Tarascon Pocket Pharmacopoeia™

2001 Classic Shirt-Pocket Edition

"Desire to take medicines ... distinguishes man from animals." *Sir William Osler*

NOTICES, TABLES, FORMULAS 2
ANALGESICS – Antirheumatics, Muscle relaxants, NSAIDs, Opioids, Other 9
ANESTHESIA – Anesthetics & Sedatives, Locals, Neuromuscular blockers 15
ANTIMICROBIALS - Aminoglycosides, Antifungals, Antimalarials, Antimycobacterials, Antiparasitics, Antivirals, Carbapenems, Cephalosporins, Macrolides, Penicillins, Quinolones, Sulfas, Tetracyclines, Other 16
CARDIOVASCULAR – ACE inhibitors, Angiotensin Receptor Blockers, Antiadrenergic agents, Antidysrhythmics, Antihyperlipidemic agents, Antihypertensives, Antiplatelet drugs, Beta blockers, Calcium channel blockers, Diuretics, Nitrates, Pressors, Thrombolytics, Volume expanders, Other 25
CONTRAST MEDIA 35
DERMATOLOGY – Acne, Antibacterials, Antifungals, Antiparasitics, Antipsoriatics, Antivirals, Corticosteroids, Hemorrhoid care, Other 35
ENDOCRINE & METABOLIC - Androgens / Anabolic Steroids, Bisphosphonates, Corticosteroids, Diabetes-related agents, Gout-Related, Minerals, Nutritionals, Thyroid agents, Vitamins, Other 41
ENT - Antihistamines, Antitussives, Decongestants, Ear preparations, ENT Combinations, Mouth and Lip preparations, Nasal preparations 47
GASTROENTEROLOGY - Antidiarrheals, Antiemetics, Antiulcer, Laxatives 51
HEMATOLOGY – Anticoagulants, Other 57
IMMUNOLOGY – Immunizations, Immunoglobulins, Immunosuppresion 58
NEUROLOGY – Alzheimer's, Anticonvulsants, Migraine, Parkinsons, Other 60
OBSTETRICS & GYNECOLOGY - Estrogens, GnRH Agonists, Hormone Replacement combos, Labor induction, Oral contraceptives, Progestins, Selective Estrogen Receptor Modulators, Tocolytics, Uterotonics, Vaginal preparations, Other 64
ONCOLOGY 69
OPHTHALMOLOGY – Antibacterials, Antivirals, Corticosteroids, Glaucoma, Mydriatics/Cycloplegics, NSAIDs, Ocular decongestants, Other 69
PSYCHIATRY – Antidepressants, Antimanics, Antipsychotics, Anxiolytics / Hypnotics, Drug dependence therapy, Sympathomimetics / Stimulants / Anorexiants, Other 70
PULMONARY – Beta agonists, Combinations, Inhaled steroids, Leukotriene inhibitors, Other 77
TOXICOLOGY 79
UROLOGY – BPH, Bladder agents, Erectile dysfunction, Nephrolithiasis, Prostate cancer, Other 80
INDEX 82
EMERGENCY DRUGS , CARDIAC DYSRHYTHMIAS, ORDERING INFO 94

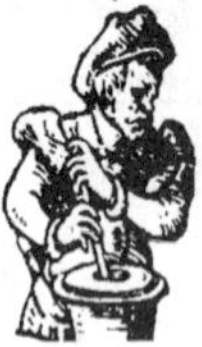

See Tarascon Publishing book ordering information on page 96.

- **Tarascon Pocket Pharmacopoeia, Classic edition**
- **Tarascon Pocket Pharmacopoeia, Deluxe edition**
- **Tarascon Internal Medicine & Critical Care Pocketbook**
- **Tarascon Adult Emergency Pocketbook**
- **Tarascon Pediatric Emergency Pocketbook**
- **How to be a Truly Excellent Junior Medical Student**

Tarascon Publishing
Box 1159
Loma Linda, CA 92354

Website: www.tarascon.com
E-mail: info@tarascon.com
Phone: (800) 929-9926

"It's not how much you know, it's how fast you can find the answer." ™

Important Caution – Please Read This!

The information in *Pocket Pharmacopoeia* is compiled from sources believed to be reliable, and exhaustive efforts have been put forth to make the book as accurate as possible. *However the accuracy and completeness of this work cannot be guaranteed*. Despite our best efforts this book may contain typographical errors and omissions. The *Pocket Pharmacopoeia* is intended as a quick and convenient reminder of information you have already learned elsewhere. The contents are to be used as a guide only, and health care professionals should use sound clinical judgment and individualize therapy to each specific patient care situation. This book is not meant to be a replacement for training, experience, continuing medical education, or studying the latest drug prescribing literature. This book is sold without warranties of any kind, express or implied, and the publisher and editors disclaim any liability, loss, or damage caused by the contents. ***If you do not wish to be bound by the foregoing cautions and conditions, you may return your undamaged and unexpired book to our office for a full refund.***

The *Tarascon Pocket Pharmacopoeia* is edited by a panel of drug information experts with extensive input from practicing clinicians of multiple specialties. Our goal is to provide health professionals focused, core prescribing information in a convenient, organized, and concise fashion. We do not include all drugs and all drug indications, but for brevity our editors have selected the most important and most common FDA-approved dosing indications as well as those off-label uses that have a reasonable basis to support their use. Tarascon Publishing is independent from and has no affiliation with pharmaceutical companies. Although drug companies purchase and distribute our books as promotional items, the Tarascon editorial staff determines all book content.

Tarascon Pocket Pharmacopoeia, *2001 Classic Edition*

ISBN 1-882742-18-4. P

HOW TO USE THE TARASCON POCKET PHARMACOPOEIA

The *Tarascon Pocket Pharmacopoeia* arranges drugs by clinical class with a comprehensive index in the back. Trade names are italicized and capitalized. Drug doses shown in mg/kg are generally intended for children, while fixed doses represent typical adult recommendations. Brackets indicate currently available formulations, although not all pharmacies stock all formulations. The availability of generic, over-the-counter, and scored formulations are mentioned. Codes are as follows:

METABOLISM & EXCRETION: **L** = primarily liver, **K** = primarily kidney, **LK** = both, but liver > kidney, **KL** = both, but kidney > liver, **LO** = liver & onions*

SAFETY IN PREGNANCY: **A** = Safety established using human studies, **B** = Presumed safety based on animal studies, **C** = Uncertain safety; no human studies and animal studies show an adverse effect, **D** = Unsafe - evidence of risk that may in certain clinical circumstances be justifiable, **X** = Highly unsafe - risk of use outweighs any possible benefit. For drugs which have not been assigned a category: **+**Generally accepted as safe, **?**Safety unknown or controversial, **-**Generally regarded as unsafe.

SAFETY IN LACTATION: **+**Generally accepted as safe, **?**Safety unknown or controversial, **-**Generally regarded as unsafe. Many of our "+" listings are taken from the AAP website (www.aap.org/policy/00026.html), and may differ from those recommended by the manufacturer.

DEA CONTROLLED SUBSTANCES: **I** = High abuse potential, no accepted use (eg, heroin, marijuana), **II** = High abuse potential and severe dependence liability (eg, morphine, codeine, hydromorphone, cocaine, amphetamines, methylphenidate, secobarbital). Some states require triplicates. **III** = Moderate dependence liability (eg, *Tylenol #3*, *Vicodin*), **IV** = Limited dependence liability (benzodiazepines, propoxyphene, phentermine), **V** = Limited abuse potential (eg, *Lomotil*).

RELATIVE COST: ***New this year!*** Clinicians are increasingly called upon to consider relative costs in drug therapy, and each of our drug entries is now coded to reflect them. The costs used (table at right) are "per month" of maintenance therapy (eg, antihypertensives) or "per course" of short-term therapy (eg, antibiotics). Codes are calculated using average wholesale prices (at press time in US dollars) for the most common indication and route of each drug at a typical adult dosage. For maintenance therapy, costs are calculated based upon a 30 day supply or the quantity that might typically be used in a given month. For short-term therapy (ie, 10 days or less), costs are calculated on a single treatment course. When multiple forms are available (eg, generics), these codes reflect the least expensive generally available product. When drugs don't neatly fit into the classification scheme above, we have assigned codes based upon the relative cost of other similar drugs. *These codes should be used as a rough guide only*, as (1) they reflect cost, not charges, (2) pricing often varies substantially from location to location and time to time, and (3) HMOs, Medicaid, and buying groups often negotiate quite different pricing. Your mileage may vary. Check with your local pharmacy if you have any question.

Code	Cost
$	< $25
$$	$25 to $49
$$$	$50 to $99
$$$$	$100 to $199
$$$$$	≥ $200

**Back by overwhelming demented demand.*

PAGE INDEX FOR TABLES*

Table	Page
General: Outpatient peds Rx	6
General: Formulas	7-8
General: Peds vitals & drugs	7
General: Therapeutic levels	8
General: Conversions	8
Analgesics: Nonsteroidals	11
Antimicrobials: STDs/Vaginitis	21
Cardiovascular: Statins	28
Dermatology: Topical steroids	38
Endocrine: Corticosteroids	42
Endocrine: Diabetes numbers	43
Endocrine: Fluoride dose	44
Endocrine: Potassium forms	45
ENT: Combination drugs	48
Gastroenterology: H pylori Rx	54
Immunology: Immunizations	59
OB/GYN: Oral contraceptives	65
OB/GYN: Drugs in pregnancy	66
Pulmonary: Peak flow	78
Pulmonary: Inhaler colors	78

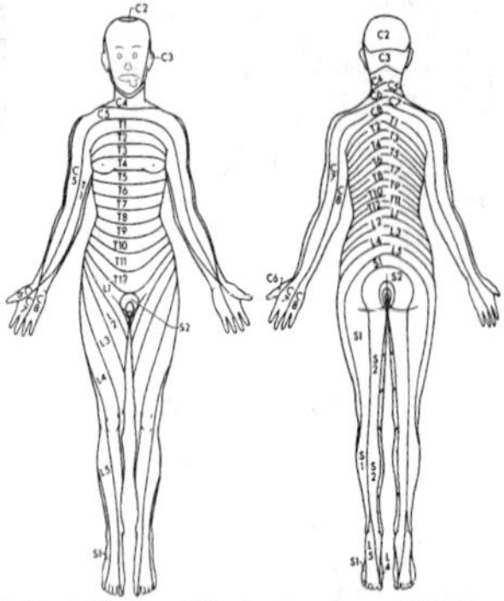

*Please see the *Pocket Pharmacopoeia Deluxe Edition* for additional tables: General: P450 Enzymes. Analgesics: Opioid equivalency. Antimicrobials: Cephalosporins, Penicillins, Quinolones, Full-length STDs/Vaginitis, Overview of bacterial pathogens; Endocarditis prophylaxis. Cardiovascular: ACE inhibitors, Cardiac parameters, Thrombolysis. Endocrine: IV solutions, peds rehydration solutions. Hematology: Oral anticoagulation. Immunology: Tetanus. Neurology: Glasgow coma scale, LS spine, Nerve roots. OB/GYN: APGAR score, Emergency contraception. Psychiatry: Body Mass Index. Pulmonary: Inhaled steroids, Asthma action plan. Toxicology: Antidotes.

ABBREVIATIONS IN TEXT

ac – before meals
ADHD – attention deficit & hyperactivity disorder
AHA – American Heart Association
ANC – absolute neutrophil count
ASA – aspirin
bid - twice per day
BPH - benign prostatic hypertrophy
cap – capsule
CMV – cytomegalovirus
CrCl – creatinine clearance
d - day
D5W - 5% dextrose
DPI – dry powder inhaler
ET - endotracheal
EPS – extrapyramidal symptoms
g - gram
gtts - drops
GERD - gastroesophageal reflux dz
GU – genitourinary
h - hour
HCTZ - hydrochlorothiazide
HRT - hormone replacement therapy
HSV – herpes simplex virus
HTN – hypertension
IM - intramuscular
INR – international normalized ratio
IU - international units
IV - intravenous
JRA - juvenile rheumatoid arthritis
kg – kilogram
LFTs – liver fxn tests
mcg - microgram
MDI – metered dose inhaler
mEq - milliequivalent
mg - milligram
MI - myocardial infarction
min - minute
mL - milliliter
mo – months old
ng - nanogram
NS - normal saline
N/V – nausea and vomiting
OA – osteoarthritis
pc – after meals
PO - by mouth
PR - by rectum
prn - as needed
q - every
qd - once daily
qhs - at bedtime
qid - four times/day
q pm – every evening
RA - rheumatoid arthritis
SC - subcutaneous
sol'n – solution
supp - suppository
susp - suspension
tab – tablet
TIA - transient ischemic attack
tid - 3 times/day
UTI – urinary tract infection
wk - week
yo - years old

If you obtained your *Pocket Pharmacopoeia* from a bookstore, please send us your address (info@tarascon.com). This allows you to be the first to know about new editions or updates! Got any ideas for improving future editions of the *Pocket Pharmacopoeia* without increasing its size? Write to us! We apologize in advance that time does not permit us to answer most inquiries. The cover woodcut is *The Apothecary* by Jost Amman, Frankfurt, 1574. Amazingly, about 10,000 of you knew off the top of your head that Ytterby, Sweden was the town that has 4 elements of the periodic tab[le] after it (terbium, ytterbium, erbium, yttrium). We will send a free copy of n[ext] edition to the first 25 who know what it will take to get Donald to return to Anna[...]

OUTPATIENT PEDIATRIC DRUGS		*Age*	*2m*	*4m*	*6m*	*9m*	*12m*	*15m*	*2y*	*3y*	*5y*
		Kg	5	6½	8	9	10	11	13	15	19
		Lbs	11	15	17	20	22	24	28	33	42
med	***strength***	***freq***	***teaspoons of liquid per dose** (1 tsp= 5 ml)*								
Tylenol (mg)		q4h	80	100	120	120	160	160	200	240	280
Tylenol (tsp)	160/t	q4h	½	½	¾	¾	1	1	1¼	1½	1¾
ibuprofen (mg)		q6h	-	-	75†	75†	100	100	125	150	175
ibuprofen (tsp)	100/t	q6h	-	-	¾†	¾†	1	1	1¼	1½	1¾
amoxicillin (bid)*	125/t	bid	1	1¼	1½	1¾	1¾	2	2¼	2¾	3½
"	250/t	bid	½	½	¾	¾	1	1	1¼	1¼	1¾
amoxicillin (tid)*	125/t	tid	½	¾	1	1	1¼	1¼	1½	1¾	2
"	250/t	tid	¼	½	½	½	¾	¾	¾	1	1
*Augmentin**	200/t	bid	½†	¾	1	1	1¼	1¼	1½	1¾	2¼
"	400/t	bid	¼†	½	½	½	¾	¾	¾	1	1
azithromycin*‡	100/t	qd	--	½†	½	½	½	½	¾	¾	1
"	200/t	qd	--	¼†	¼	¼	¼	¼	½	½	½
Bactrim/Septra	---	bid	½	¾	1	1	1	1¼	1½	1½	2
cefaclor*	125/t	bid	--	1†	1¼†	1½	1½	1¾	2	2½	3
"	250/t	bid	--	½†	¾†	¾	¾	1	1	1¼	1½
cefadroxil	125/t	bid	½	¾	1	1	1¼	1¼	1½	1¾	2
"	250/t	bid	¼	½	½	½	¾	¾	¾	1	1
cefdinir	125/t	qd	--	¾†	1	1	1	1¼	1½	1¾	2
cefixime	100/t	qd	--	½	¾	¾	1	1	1¼	1¼	1½
cefprozil*	125/t	bid	--	¾†	1	1	1¼	1½	1½	2	2¼
"	250/t	bid	--	½†	½	½	¾	¾	¾	1	1¼
cephalexin	125/t	qid	--	½†	¾†	¾†	1	1	1¼	1½	1¾
"	250/t	qid	--	¼†	¼†	½†	½	½	¾	¾	1
clarithromycin	125/t	bid	--	½†	½†	½	¾	¾	¾	1	1¼
"	250/t	bid	--	¼†	¼†	¼	½	½	½	½	¾
dicloxacillin	62½/t	qid	½	¾	1	1	1¼	1¼	1½	1¾	2
loracarbef*	100/t	bid	--	1†	1¼	1½	1½	1¾	2	2¼	3
Pediazole	---	tid	½	½	¾	¾	1	1	1	1¼	1½
penicillin	125/t	qid	½	½	¾	¾	1	1	1¼	1¼	1½
"	250/t	qid	--	¼	¼	½	½	½	¾	¾	1
Benadryl	12.5/t	q6h	½	½	¾	¾	1	1	1¼	1½	2
Dimetapp	---	q4h	-		¼†	¼†	½	½	¾	¾	1
prednisone	5/t	qd	1	1¼	1½	1¾	2	2¼	2½	3	3¾
Robitussin	---	q4h	-	-	¼†	¼†	½	½	¾	¾	1
Rondec	---	q4h	-	-	-	-	¼†	¼†	½	½	1
Triaminic	---	q4h	-	¼	¼	¼	½	½	1	1	1
Tylenol w/ Codeine		q4h	-	-	-	-	-	-	-	1	1
Ventolin	2/t	tid	-	-	-	-	½	½	¾	¾	1

* Dose shown is for otitis media only; see dosing in text for alternative indications.

† Dosing at this age/weight not recommended by manufacturer.

Give a double dose of azithromycin the first day.

PEDIATRIC VITAL SIGNS AND INTRAVENOUS DRUGS

Age		Pre-matr	New-born	2m	4m	6m	9m	12m	15m	2y	3y	5y
Weight	(Kg)	2	3½	5	6½	8	9	10	11	13	15	19
	(Lbs)	4½	7½	11	15	17	20	22	24	28	33	42
Maint fluids	(ml/h)	8	14	20	26	32	36	40	42	46	50	60
ET tube	(mm)	2½	3	3½	3½	3½	4	4	4½	4½	4½	5
Defib	(Joules)	4	7	10	13	10	18	20	22	26	30	38
Systolic BP	(high)	70	80	90	100	110	110	120	120	120	120	120
	(low)	50	60	70	70	70	70	70	70	70	70	70
Pulse rate	(high)	145	145	180	180	180	160	160	160	150	150	135
	(low)	100	100	110	110	110	100	100	100	90	90	65
Resp rate	(high)	45	45	45	40	35	35	30	30	30	24	24
	(low)	35	35	35	30	25	25	20	20	20	16	14
epinephrine	(mg)	.02	.04	.05	.07	.08	.09	0.1	0.11	0.13	0.15	0.19
atropine	(mg)	0.1	0.1	0.1	0.14	0.16	0.18	0.2	0.22	0.26	0.30	0.38
bicarbonate	(meq)	2	3½	5	6½	8	9	10	11	13	15	19
lidocaine	(mg)	2	3½	5	6½	8	9	10	11	13	15	19
Benadryl	(mg)	-	-	5	6½	8	9	10	11	13	15	19
dextrose	(g)	2	3½	5	6½	8	9	10	11	13	15	19
morphine	(mg)	0.2	0.3	0.5	0.6	0.8	0.9	1	1.1	1.3	1.5	1.9
mannitol	(g)	2	3½	5	6½	8	9	10	11	13	15	19
diazepam	(mg)	0.6	1	1.5	2	2.5	2.7	3	3.3	3.9	4.5	5
lorazepam	(mg)	0.1	0.2	0.3	0.35	0.4	0.5	0.5	0.6	0.7	0.8	1.0
phenobarb	(mg)	30	60	75	100	125	125	150	175	200	225	275
ceftriaxone	(mg)	-	-	250	325	400	450	500	550	650	750	1000
cefotaxime	(mg)	100	175	250	325	400	450	500	550	650	750	1000
ampicillin	(mg)	100	175	250	325	400	450	500	550	650	750	1000
gentamicin	(mg)	6	7	10	13	16	18	20	22	26	30	38

Alveolar-arterial oxygen gradient = A-a = 148 - 1.2(PaCO2) - PaO2
[normal = 10-20 mmHg, breathing room air at sea level]

Anion gap = Na – (Cl + HC03) [normal = 10-14 meq/L]

Calculated osmolality = 2Na + glucose/18 + BUN/2.8 + ethanol/4.6 + isopropanol/6 + methanol/3.2 + ethylene-glycol/6.2 [norm 280-295]

Golden rules of arterial blood gases

1) PCO_2 increase of 10 corresponds to a pH drop of 0.08.
2) pH drop of 0.15 corresponds to base excess decrease of 10 meq/l.

Pediatric IV maintenance fluids (see table above):

4 ml/kg/hr **or** 100 ml/kg/day for first 10 kg, plus
2 ml/kg/hr **or** 50 ml/kg/day for second 10 kg, plus
1 ml/kg/hr **or** 20 ml/kg/day for all further kg

THERAPEUTIC DRUG LEVELS

Drug	Level	Optimal Timing
amikacin peak	20-35 mcg/ml	1 hour after start of 30-60 min infusion
amikacin trough	<5 mcg/ml	Just prior to next dose
carbamazepine trough	4-12 mcg/ml	Just prior to next dose
cyclosporine trough	50-300 ng/ml	Just prior to next dose
digoxin	0.8-2.2 ng/ml	Just prior to next dose
ethosuximide trough	40-100 mcg/ml	Just prior to next dose
gentamicin peak	5-10 mcg/ml	1 hour after start of 30-60 min infusion
gentamicin trough	<2 mcg/ml	Just prior to next dose
lidocaine	1-5 mcg/ml	4-8 hours after start of infusion
lithium trough	0.6-1.2 meq/l	Just prior to first morning dose
NAPA	10-30 mcg/ml	Just prior to next procainamide dose
phenobarbital trough	15-40 mcg/ml	Just prior to next dose
phenytoin trough	10-20 mcg/ml	Just prior to next dose
primidone trough	5-12 mcg/ml	Just prior to next dose
procainamide	4-8 mcg/ml	Just prior to next dose
quinidine	1-4 mcg/ml	Just prior to next dose
theophylline	5-15 mcg/ml	8-12 hrs after once daily dose
tobramycin peak	5-10 mcg/ml	1 hour after start of 30-60 min infusion
tobramycin trough	<2 mcg/ml	Just prior to next dose
valproic acid trough	50-100 mcg/ml	Just prior to next dose
vancomycin trough	5-10 mcg/ml	Just prior to next dose

$$\text{mcg/kg/min} = \frac{16.7 \times \text{Drug Conc [mg/ml]} \times \text{Infusion Rate [ml/h]}}{\text{Weight [kg]}}$$

$$\text{Infusion rate [ml/h]} = \frac{\text{Desired mcg/kg/min} \times \text{Weight [kg]} \times 60}{\text{Drug concentration [mcg/ml]}}$$

Fractional excression of sodium = [Pre-renal <1%, renal (ATN) >1%]

$$\left[\frac{\text{urine Na / plasma Na}}{\text{urine creat / plasma creat}}\right] \times 100\%$$

Creatinine clearance [normal >80]

$$= \frac{(\text{lean kg})(140 - \text{age})(0.85 \text{ if female})}{(72)(\text{stable creatinine})}$$

Body surface area (BSA) [in m^2] = square root of:

$$\left[\frac{\text{height (cm)} \times \text{weight (kg)}}{3600}\right]$$

CONVERSIONS	*Liquid:*	*Weight:*
Temperature:	1 fluid ounce = 30ml	1 kilogram = 2.2 lbs
F = (1.8) C + 32	1 teaspoon = 5ml	1 ounce = 30 g
C = (F - 32)/(1.8)	1 tablespoon = 15ml	1 grain = 65 mg

ANALGESICS

Antirheumatic Agents

auranofin (*Ridaura*): RA: 3mg PO bid or 6mg qd, max 3mg tid. [Trade: Caps 3mg.] ▶K ♀C ▶- $$$$

aurothioglucose (*Solganal*): RA: first week 10mg IM, doses increase weekly to 50mg. ▶K ♀C ▶- $$$$$

azathioprine (*Imuran*): RA: initial dose 1mg/kg (50-100mg) PO qd or divided bid. Increase after 6-8 weeks. [Generic/Trade: Tabs 50mg, scored.] ▶LK ♀D ▶- $$$

etanercept (*Enbrel*): RA: 25mg SC 2X/week. JRA 4-17 yo: 0.4mg/kg SC 2X/week, to max single dose of 25mg. [Supplied in 4 dose tray carton.] ▶K ♀B ▶- $$$$$

gold sodium thiomalate (*Aurolate*): RA: first week 10mg IM, doses increase weekly to 50mg ▶K ♀C ▶- $$$$$

hydroxychloroquine sulfate (*Plaquenil*): RA: start 400-600mg PO qd, then taper to 200-400mg qd. SLE: 400 PO qd/bid to start, then taper to 200-400mg qd. [Generic/Trade: Tabs 200mg, scored.] ▶K ♀C ▶? $$$$

leflunomide (*Arava*): RA: 100mg PO qd X 3; then 10-20mg PO qd. [Trade: Tabs 10, 20, & 100mg.] ▶LK ♀X ▶- $$$$$

methotrexate (*Rheumatrex*): RA: Start with 7.5mg/week PO single dose or 2.5mg PO q12h X 3 doses given as a course once weekly. Max dose 20mg/week. Supplement with 1mg/day of folic acid. [Generic/Trade: Tabs 2.5mg, scored.] ▶LK ♀X ▶- $

sulfasalazine (*Azulfidine, Azulfidine EN-tabs, Salazopyrin EN-Tabs, S.A.S.*): RA: 500mg PO qd/bid after meals up to 1g PO bid. May turn body fluids, contact lenses or skin orange-yellow. [Generic/Trade: Tabs 500mg, scored; Trade only: Enteric Coated (EN-Tabs) 500mg.] ▶LK ♀B ▶- $

Muscle Relaxants

baclofen (*Lioresal*): Spasticity related to MS or spinal cord disease/injury: Start 5mg PO tid, then increase by 5mg/dose every 3 days until 20mg PO tid. Max dose 20mg qid. [Generic/Trade: Tabs 10 & 20mg, trade scored.] ▶K ♀C ▶? $

carisoprodol (*Soma*): Musculoskeletal pain: 350mg PO tid/qid. Abuse potential. [Generic/Trade:Tabs 350mg.] ▶LK ♀? ▶- $

chlorzoxazone (*Paraflex, Parafon Forte DSC, Remular-S*): Musculoskeletal pain: 500-750mg PO tid/qid to start; decrease to 250mg tid/qid. [Generic/Trade:Tabs & caplets 250 & 500mg (Parafon Forte DSC 500mg caplets scored).] ▶LK ♀? ▶? $

cyclobenzaprine (*Flexeril*): Musculoskeletal pain: Start 10mg PO tid, max 60mg/day. Not recommended in elderly. [Generic/Trade: Tabs 10mg.] ▶LK ♀B ▶? $

diazepam (*Valium, Diastat*): Skeletal muscle spasm, spasticity: 2-10mg PO tid/qid. [Generic/Trade: Tabs 2, 5 & 10mg, trade scored; Generic: Oral sol'n 5mg/5ml & 5mg/ml (Intensol)] ▶LK ♀D ▶- ©IV $

metaxalone (*Skelaxin*): Musculoskeletal pain: 800mg PO tid/qid. [Trade: Tabs 400mg, scored.] ▶LK ♀? ▶? $$

methocarbamol (*Robaxin, Robaxin-750*): Acute musculoskeletal pain: 1,500mg PO qid or 1,000mg IM/IV tid X 48-72h. Maintenance: 1,000mg PO qid, 750mg PO q4h, or 1,500mg PO tid. [Generic/Trade: Tabs 500 & 750mg. OTC in Canada.] ▶LK ♀C ▶+ $

orphenadrine (*Norflex*): Musculoskeletal pain: 100mg PO bid 60mg IV/IM bid. [Generic: Tabs 100mg; Generic/Trade: 100mg sust'd release. OTC in Canada.] ▶LK ♀C ▶

quinine sulfate: Commonly prescribed for nocturnal leg cramps, but not FDA approved for this indication: 260-325mg PO hs. Cinchonism with overdose; hemolysis with G-6PD deficiency, hypersensitivity. [Rx only: Generic: Caps 200, 260 & 325mg; Tabs 260mg.] ▶L ♀X ▶? $

tizanidine (*Zanaflex*): Muscle spasticity due to MS or spinal cord injury: 4-8mg PO q6-8h prn, max 36mg/d. [Trade: Tabs 4mg, scored.] ▶LK ♀C ▶? $$$$

Non-Opioid Analgesic Combinations

Ascriptin (ASA with Mg/Al hydroxide & Ca carbonate buffers): Multiple strengths; write specific product on Rx. 1-2 tabs PO q4h. [Trade: Tabs *Ascriptin A/D* aspirin 325mg, *Ascriptin Maximum Strength* aspirin 500mg.] ▶K ♀D ▶? $

Esgic, Fioricet (acetaminophen/butalbital/caffeine): 1-2 tabs PO q4h. [Generic/Trade: Tabs acetaminophen 325mg/butalbital 50mg/caffeine 40mg.] ▶LK ♀C ▶? $

Fiorinal (ASA/butalbital/caffeine): 1-2 tabs PO q4h. [Generic/Trade: Tabs aspirin 325mg/butalbital 50mg/caffeine 40mg.] ▶KL ♀D ▶- ©III $

Norgesic (orphenadrine/ASA/caffeine): Multiple strengths; write specific product on Rx. Norgesic, 1-2 tabs PO tid/qid. Norgesic Forte, 1 tab PO tid/qid. [Trade: Tabs Norgesic 25/385/30 mg, Norgesic Forte 50/770/60 mg.] ▶KL ♀D ▶? $$$

Robaxisal (methocarbamol/ASA): 2 tabs PO qid. [Generic/Trade: Tabs methocarbamol 400mg/ASA 325mg.] ▶LK ♀D ▶? $

Soma Compound (carisoprodol/ASA): 1-2 tabs PO qid. [Generic/Trade: Tabs carisoprodol 200mg/ASA 325 mg.] ▶LK ♀D ▶- $$

Nonsteroidal Anti-Inflammatories

NOTE: All NSAIDs are pregnancy class D in the 3rd trimester. Chronic use may precipitate renal insufficiency, gastritis, peptic ulcer disease, and GI bleeds. Caution in liver disease.

Arthrotec (diclofenac/misoprostol): OA: one 50/200 PO tid. RA: one 50/200 PO tid-qid. If intolerant, may use 50/200 or 75/200 PO bid. Misoprostol is an abortifacient. [Trade: Tabs 50mg/200mcg & 75mg/200mcg.] ▶LK ♀X ▶- $$$$

aspirin (*Ecotrin, Empirin, Bayer, ASA, Asaphen*): 325-650mg PO/PR q4-6h. [OTC: Tabs 81, 165, 325, 500, 650, controlled release Tabs 650 (scored). Rx only: 800mg controlled release Tabs & 975mg enteric coated; OTC: supp 120, 200, 300, & 600mg.] ▶K ♀D ▶? $

celecoxib (*Celebrex*): OA: 200mg PO qd or 100mg PO bid. RA: 100mg - 200mg PO bid; familial adenomatous polyposis: 400mg PO bid with food. Contraindicated in sulfonamide allergy. [Trade: Caps 100 & 200mg.] ▶L ♀C ▶? $$$

diclofenac (*Voltaren, Voltaren XR, Cataflam*): Multiple strengths; write specific product on Rx. Immediate or delayed release 50mg PO bid/tid or 75mg PO bid. Extended release (Voltaren XR): 100-200mg PO qd. [Generic/Trade: Tabs, immediate release (bid-tid) 50mg; Tabs, delayed release (bid-tid) 25, 50, & 75mg; Trade only: Tabs, extended release (qd) (Voltaren XR) 100mg.] ▶L ♀B ▶- $$$

diflunisal (*Dolobid*): 500-1000mg initially, then 250-500mg PO q8-12h. [Generic/Trade: Tabs 250 & 500mg.] ▶K ♀C ▶- $$$

etodolac (*Lodine, Lodine XL, Ultradol*): Multiple strengths; specify specific product. Immediate release 200-400mg PO bid/tid. Ext release (Lodine XL): 400-1200mg PO qd. [Generic/Trade: Tabs, immediate release (bid-qid) 400mg. Trade only: Caps, immed. release (bid-tid) 200,300mg; Tabs, ext release (qd) 400,500,600mg.] ▶L ♀C ▶- $$$

NONSTEROIDALS – If one class fails, consider another. *Salicylates*: aspirin, salsalate, diflunisal. *Propionic acids*: flurbiprofen, ibuprofen, ketoprofen, naproxen, oxaprozin. *Acetic acids*: diclofenac, etodolac, indomethacin, ketorolac, nabumetone, sulindac, tolmetin. *Fenamates*: meclofenamate. *Oxicams*: meloxicam, piroxicam. *COX-2 inhibitors*: celecoxib, rofecoxib.

flurbiprofen (*Ansaid, Froben*): 200-300mg/day PO divided bid-qid. [Generic/Trade: Tabs immediate release 50 & 100mg.] ▶L ♀B ▶+ $$$

ibuprofen (*Motrin, Advil, Nuprin, Rufen*): 200-800mg PO tid-qid. Peds >6 mo: 5-10 mg/kg PO q6-8h. [OTC: Caps, 200mg; Tabs 100, 200mg; Chewable Tabs 50 & 100 mg; Caplets 200mg; Liquid & susp, 100mg/5ml, susp 100mg/2.5ml; infant drops, 50 mg/1.25ml (Calibrated dropper). Rx only: Tabs 400, 600 & 800mg.] ▶L ♀D ▶+ $

indomethacin (*Indocin, Indocin SR, Indocid, Indotec*): Multiple strengths; specify specific product. Immediate release 25-50mg cap or supp PO/PR tid. Sust'd release: 75 mg cap PO qd/bid. [Generic/Trade: Immediate release (tid-qid) Caps 25 & 50mg; oral susp 25mg/5ml; supp 50mg; Trade only: sust'd release (qd-bid) 75mg.] ▶L ♀? ▶+ $

ketoprofen (*Orudis, Actron, Oruvail, Orafen*): Immediate release: 25-75mg PO tid/qid. Extended release (Oruvail): 100-200mg cap PO qd. [OTC: Tabs immediate release, 12.5mg. Rx, Trade only immediate release: Caps 25, 50 & 75mg; Caps, extended release (qd) (Oruvail) 100, 150mg; Rx, Generic/Trade: Caps, extended release (qd) & 200mg.] ▶L ♀B ▶- $$$

ketorolac (*Toradol*): Moderately severe acute pain,15-30mg IV/IM q6h or 10mg tab PO q4-6h prn; combined duration IV/IM and PO is not to exceed 5 days. [Generic/Trade: Tabs 10mg.] ▶L ♀C ▶+ $

meclofenamate: 50-100mg cap PO tid/qid. [Generic: Caps immediate release: 50 & 100mg.] ▶L ♀? ▶- $$$$$

meloxicam (*Mobic*): OA: 7.5mg tab PO qd. [Trade: Tabs, 7.5 mg] ▶L ♀C ▶? $$$

nabumetone (*Relafen*): RA/OA: Starting dose: 500mg tab x 2 (1000mg) PO qd. May increase to 1500-2000mg tab(s) PO qd or divided bid. [Trade: Tabs 500 & 750mg.] ▶L ♀C ▶- $$$

naproxen (*Naprosyn, Aleve, Anaprox, EC-Naprosyn, Naprelan, Naxen, Synflex*): Immediate release: 250-500mg PO bid. Delayed release: 375-500mg PO bid. Controlled release: 750-1000mg PO qd. JRA: ≤13kg 2.5ml PO bid; 14-25kg 5ml PO bid, 26-38kg 7.5ml PO bid. [OTC, Generic/Trade: Tabs immed release (bid-tid) 200mg; Rx only, Generic/Trade: Tabs immed (bid) 250, 375 & 500mg; Rx, Trade only: Tabs, del'd release (bid), enteric coated [do not crush or chew], 375 & 500mg; Tabs, cont'l release 375 & 500mg (qd); immed release susp (bid-tid)125mg/5ml.] ▶L ♀B ▶- $$$

oxaprozin (*Daypro*): 1200mg PO qd. [Generic/Trade: Caplets 600mg, trade scored.] ▶L ♀C ▶- $$$

piroxicam (*Feldene, Fexicam*): 20mg cap PO qd. [Generic/Trade: Caps 10 & 20mg.] ▶L ♀? ▶+ $$$

rofecoxib (*Vioxx*): OA: 12.5-25mg PO qd; Acute pain, dysmenorrhea: 50mg PO qd. [Trade: Tabs 12.5,25,50 mg; susp 12.5mg/5ml and 25mg/5ml.] ▶Plasma ♀C ▶? $$$

salsalate (*Salflex, Disalcid*): 3000mg/day PO divided q8-12h. [Generic/Trade: Tabs 500 & 750mg, various scored; Trade only: Caps 500mg.] ▶K ♀C ▶? $$

sulindac (*Clinoril*): 150-200mg tab PO bid [Generic/Trade: Immediate release Tabs 150 & 200mg.] ▶L ♀? ▶- $$$

tolmetin (*Tolectin*): 200-600mg PO tid. [Generic/Trade: Tabs immediate release 200 (trade scored) & 600mg; Caps immediate release 400mg.] ▸L ♀C ▸+ $$$

Trilisate (choline/magnesium salicylate): 1500mg PO bid. [Generic/Trade: Immediate release Tabs 500, 750, & 1000mg, scored; liquid 500mg/5ml.] ▸K ♀C ▸? $$$

Opioid Agonist-Antagonists (see also combination analgesics)

buprenorphine (*Buprenex*): 0.3-0.6mg IV/IM q6-8h prn. ▸L ♀C ▸? ©V $$

butorphanol (*Stadol, Stadol NS*): 0.5-2mg IV or 1-4mg IM q3-4h prn. Nasal spray (Stadol NS): 1 spray q3-4h. Abuse potential. [Nasal spray 1mg/spray, 2.5ml bottle (14-15 doses/bottle).] ▸LK ♀C ▸+ ©IV $$$

dezocine (*Dalgan*): 2.5-10mg IV q2-4h or 5-20mg IM q3-6h prn. ▸LK ♀C ▸- $

nalbuphine (*Nubain*): 10-20mg IV/IM/SC q3-6h. ▸LK ♀? ▸? $

pentazocine (*Talwin, Talwin NX*): 30mg IV/IM q3-4h prn (Talwin); 1 tab PO q3-4h. (Talwin NX -pentazocine 50mg/naloxone 0.5mg). [Generic/Trade: Tabs 50mg with 0.5mg naloxone, trade scored.] ▸LK ♀C ▸? ©IV $

Opioid Agonists

NOTE: Patients with chronic pain may require more frequent and higher dosing. Opioids commonly create constipation. All opioids are pregnancy class D if used for prolonged periods or in high doses at term. May cause drowsiness and/or sedation.

codeine: 0.5mg/kg up to 15-60mg PO/IM/IV/SC q4-6h. Do not use IV in children. [Generic: Tabs 15, 30, & 60mg; Oral sol'n: 15mg/5 ml.] ▸LK ♀C ▸+ ©II $

fentanyl (*Duragesic Patches, Actiq, Fentanyl Oralet*): Transdermal (Duragesic): 1 patch q72 hrs (some chronic pain pts may req q48h dosing). Transmucosal lozenge for breakthrough cancer pain (Actiq): 200-1,600mcg; max dose 4 lozenges on a stick/ day; premedication in a hospital setting (Oralet): 5-15mcg/kg up to 400mcg as a max single dose. [Trade: Transdermal patches 25, 50, 75, & 100mcg/h (Duragesic). Multiple patches may be used if needed. Transmucosal forms: lozenges on a stick, raspberry flavored 200, 400, 600, 800, 1,200, & 1,600mcg (Actiq lozenges on a stick); 100,200, 300,400mcg (Fentanyl Oralet lozenges).] ▸L ♀C ▸? ©II $$$$$

hydromorphone (*Dilaudid, Dilaudid-5*): 2-4mg PO q4-6h. Titrate dose as high as necessary to relieve pain requiring chronic opioids. 0.5-2mg IM/SC or slow IV q4-6h. 3mg PR q6-8h. [Generic/Trade: Tabs 2, 4, & 8mg (8mg trade scored); liquid 5mg/5ml (Dilaudid); supp 3mg. Trade only: Tabs 1 & 3mg.] ▸L ♀C ▸? ©II $$$

levorphanol (*Levo-Dromoran*): 2mg PO/SC q6-8h. [Trade: Tabs 2mg, scored.] ▸L ♀C ▸? ©II $$$

meperidine (*Demerol*): 1-1.8mg/kg up to 150mg IM/SC/PO or slow IV q3-4h. Conversion 75mg IV,IM,SC = 300mg PO [Generic/Trade:Tabs 50 (trade scored) & 100mg; syrup 50mg/5ml (trade banana flavored).] ▸LK ♀C but + ▸- ©II $

methadone (*Dolophine, Methadose*): Severe pain: 2.5-10mg IM/SC/PO q3-4h prn. Titrate dose as high as necessary to relieve pain requiring chronic opioids. Detoxification: 15-40mg PO qd to start, then decrease by 20% q1-2 days. [Generic/Trade: Tabs 5, 10, various scored; oral concentrate: 10mg/ml; dispersible Tabs 40mg; Generic only: oral sol'n 5 & 10mg/5ml.] ▸L ♀C ▸? ©II $$$

morphine sulfate (*MS Contin, Kadian, Roxanol, Oramorph SR, MSIR, Statex*): 10-30mg PO q4h (immediate release tabs, caps, supp, or oral sol'n). Controlled-release tabs (MS Contin, Oramorph SR): 30mg PO q8-12h. Controlled release caps (Kadian): 20

mg PO q12h. Do not break, chew, or crush controlled release preparations. Do not open Kadian caps; they must be swallowed whole. 0.1-0.2mg/kg up to 15mg IM/SC or slow IV q4h. Titrate dose as high as necessary to relieve pain requiring chronic opioids. [Generic/Trade: Immediate release: Tabs 15 & 30mg; Trade: Caps 15 & 30 mg; Immediate release. Generic/Trade: oral sol'n (Roxanol) 10mg/5ml, 10mg/2.5ml, 20mg/5ml, 20mg/ml (concentrate) & 100mg/5ml (concentrate) & rectal supp 5, 10, 20 & 30mg. Controlled release Tabs (q12h some pts require q8h) (MS Contin, Oramorph SR) 15, 30, 60, 100 & (200mg MS Contin Only); Controlled release Caps (q24h or q12h - do not give q8h) (Kadian) 20, 50 & 100 mg.] ▶L ♀C ▶+ ©II $$$$

oxycodone (*Roxicodone, OxyContin, Percolone, OxyIR, OxyFAST, Endocodone, Supeudol*): Immediate release preparations: 5mg PO q6h prn. Controlled release (OxyContin): 10-40mg PO q12h (No supporting data for shorter dosing intervals for controlled release tabs.) Titrate dose as high as necessary to relieve pain requiring chronic opioids. Do not break/chew/crush controlled release preps. [Trade: Immed release: Tabs (scored) & Caps 5mg; oral sol'n 5mg/5ml; oral concentrate 20mg/ml. Controlled release Tabs q12h (OxyContin): 10,20,40,80,160mg.] ▶L ♀C ▶- ©II $$$$

oxymorphone (*Numorphan*): 1-1.5mg IM/SC q4-6h prn. 0.5mg IV initial dose in healthy patients patients then q4-6h prn, increase dose until pain adequately controlled. 5mg PR q4-6h prn. [Trade only: supp 5mg.] ▶L ♀C ▶? ©II $

propoxyphene (*Darvon-N, Darvon Pulvules*): 65mg PO q4h prn. [Generic/Trade: Caps 65mg; Trade only: 100mg (Darvon-N).] ▶L ♀C ▶+ ©IV $

Opioid Analgesic Combinations

NOTE: The maximum adult daily dose of acetaminophen should not exceed 4g. Opioids commonly create constipation. All opioids are pregnancy class D if used for prolonged periods or in high doses at term. May cause drowsiness and/or sedation.

Anexsia (hydrocodone/acetaminophen): Multiple strengths; specify product. 1 tab PO q4-6h prn. [Generic/Trade: Tabs 5/500, 7.5/650, 10/660mg, scored.] ▶LK ♀+ ▶- ©III $

Capital with Codeine susp (acetaminophen/codeine): 15ml PO q4h prn; >12yo use adult dose, 7-12 yo 10ml/dose q4-6h prn, 3-6 yo 5ml/dose q4-6h prn. [Generic: oral sol'n; Trade: susp: codeine 12mg/acetaminophen 120mg/5ml (trade, fruit punch flavor).] ▶LK ♀C ▶? ©V $

Darvocet (propoxyphene/acetaminophen): Multiple strengths; specify product. 50/325, 2 tabs PO q4h prn; 100/650, 1 tab PO q4h prn. [Generic/Trade: Tabs 50/325mg (Darvocet N-50) & 100/650 mg (Darvocet N-100)] ▶L ♀C ▶? ©IV $

Darvon Compound-65 Pulvules (propoxyphene/ASA/caffeine): 1 cap PO q4h prn. [Generic/Trade: Caps, 65 propoxyphene/389 ASA/32.4 caffeine mg.] ▶LK ♀D ▶- ©IV $

Empirin with Codeine (ASA/codeine): Multiple strengths; specify product.1-2 tabs PO q4h prn. [Generic/Trade: Tabs 325/30mg (Empirin with codeine #3) & 325mg/60 (Empirin with codeine #4), ASA/codeine.] ▶LK ♀D ▶- ©III $

Fioricet with Codeine (acetaminophen/butalbital/caffeine/codeine): 1-2 caps PO q4h prn. [Trade: Caps, 325/50/40/30 mg.] ▶LK ♀C ▶- ©III $$$

Fiorinal with Codeine (ASA/butalbital/caffeine/codeine): 1-2 caps PO q4h prn. [Trade: Caps, ASA 325/50/40/30 mg.] ▶LK ♀D ▶- ©III $$$

Lorcet (hydrocodone/acetaminophen): Multiple strengths. 5/500: 1-2 tabs PO q4-6h prn. 7.5/650 & 10/650: 1 tab PO q4-6h prn. [Generic/Trade: Caps, Lorcet HD (5/500); Tabs, Lorcet Plus (7.5/650); Trade: (Lorcet -10/650), scored.] ▶LK ♀+ ▶- ©III $

Lortab (hydrocodone/acetaminophen): Multiple strengths; specify product. 1-2 tabs PO q4-6h prn (2.5/500 & 5/500). 1 tab PO q4-6h prn (7.5/500 & 10/500). Elixir: 15ml PO q4-6h prn. [Trade: Tabs Lortab 2.5/500; Generic/Trade: Lortab 5/500 (scored), Lortab 7.5/500 (trade scored) & Lortab 10/500mg, hydrocodone/acetaminophen; Trade only: Lortab Elixir: 7.5/500mg hydrocodone/acetaminophen per 15ml.] ▶LK ♀+ ◗- ©III $

Norco (hydrocodone/acetaminophen): 1 tab PO q4-6h prn; max 6/day. [Trade: Tabs: 10mg hydrocodone/ 325mg acetaminophen, scored.] ▶L ♀C ◗? ©III $$

Percocet (oxycodone/acetaminophen): Multiple strengths; specify product. 1-2 tabs PO q6h prn (2.5/325 & 5/325). 1 tab PO q6 prn (7.5/500 & 10/650). [Trade: Tabs Percocet 2.5/325, Percocet 7.5/500, Percocet 10/650; Generic/Trade: Tabs Percocet 5mg/325mg, oxycodone/acetaminophen.] ▶L ♀C ◗- ©II $

Percodan (oxycodone/ASA): 1 tab PO q6h prn (5/325mg); 1-2 tabs PO q6h prn (2.5/325). [Generic/Trade: Tabs Perodan 5/325 (trade scored); Trade only: 2.5/325 mg (Percodan Demi) scored, oxycodone/ASA.] ▶LK ♀D ◗- ©II $

Roxicet (oxycodone/acetaminophen): Multiple strengths; specify product. 1 tab PO q6h prn. Sol'n: 5ml PO q6h prn. [Generic/Trade: Tablet Roxicet 5/325mg, scored; Caplet Roxicet 5/500mg, scored; Trade only: Roxicet oral sol'n 5/325mg per 5ml, oxycodone/acetaminophen.] ▶L ♀C ◗- ©II $

Soma Compound with Codeine (carisoprodol/ASA/codeine): Moderate to severe musculoskeletal pain:1-2 tabs PO qid prn. [Trade: Tabs carisoprodol 200mg/ASA 325mg/codeine 16mg.] ▶L ♀C ◗- ©III $$$

Talacen (pentazocine/acetaminophen): 1 tab PO q4h prn. [Trade: Tabs pentazocine 25mg/acetaminophen 650mg, scored.] ▶L ♀C ◗? ©IV $$$

Tylenol with Codeine (codeine/acetaminophen): Multiple strengths; specify product. 1-2 tabs PO q4h prn. Elixir 3-6 yo 5ml/dose, 7-12 yo 10ml/dose q4-6h prn. [Generic/ Trade: Tabs Tylenol #2 (15/300)), Tylenol #3 (30/300), Tylenol #4 (60/300); Tylenol with Codeine Elixir 12mg/120mg per 5ml] ▶LK ♀C ◗? ©III (Tabs), V(elixir) $

Tylox (oxycodone/acetaminophen): 1 cap PO q6h prn. [Generic/Trade: Caps, oxycodone 5mg/acetaminophen 500mg.] ▶L ♀C ◗- ©II $

Vicodin (hydrocodone/acetaminophen): Multiple strengths; specify product. 5/500 (max dose 8 tabs/day) & 7.5/750 (max dose of 5 tabs/day), 1-2 tabs PO q4-6h prn; 10/660 1 tab PO q4-6h prn (max of 6 tabs/day). [Generic/Trade: Tabs Vicodin (5/500mg), Vicodin ES (7.5/750), Vicodin HP (10/660mg), scored;] ▶LK ♀+ ◗? ©III $

Vicoprofen (hydrocodone/ibuprofen): 1-2 tabs PO q4h prn. [Trade: Tabs hydrocodone 7.5mg/ibuprofen 200mg.] ▶LK ♀- ◗? ©III $$$

Wygesic (propoxyphene/acetaminophen): 1 tab PO q4h prn. [Generic/Trade: Tabs propoxyphene 65mg/acetaminophen 650mg.] ▶L ♀C ◗? ©IV $

Zydone (hydrocodone/acetaminophen): Multiple strengths; specify product. 1-2 tabs PO q4-6h prn [5/400] 1 tab q4-6h prn [7.5/400,10/400]. [Trade: Tabs (5mg/400mg), (7.5mg/400mg) & (10mg/400mg), hydrocodone/acetaminophen.] ▶LK ♀+ ◗? ©III $$

Opioid Antagonists

nalmefene (*Revex*): Opioid overdose: 0.5mg/70kg IV. If needed, give second dose of 1mg/70kg, 2-5 mins later. Max cumulative dose 1.5mg/70kg. If suspicion of opioid dependency, initially administer a challenge dose of 0.1mg/70kg. Post-operative opioid reversal: 0.25mcg/kg IV followed by 0.25mcg/kg incremental doses at 2-5 min intervals prn. Max cumulative dose 1mcg/kg. ▶L ♀B ◗? $$$

naloxone (*Narcan*): Opioid overdose: 0.4-2.0mg q2-3min prn; Adult post op reversal 0.1-0.2mg; Ped post-op reversal: 0.005-0.01mg. IV/IM/SC/FT. ▸LK ♀B ▸? $

Other Analgesics

acetaminophen (*Tylenol, Panadol, Tempra, Atasol*): 325-650mg PO/PR q4-6h prn. OA: 2 caplets (ext rel) PO q8h around the clock. Peds: 10-15mg/kg/dose PO/PR q4-6h prn. [OTC: Tabs 160, 325, 500, 650mg; chewable Tabs 80mg; gelcaps 500mg; Caps 325 & 500mg; sprinkle Caps 80 & 160mg; extended release (q8h) caplets 650mg; liquid 80mg/2.5 ml, 80, 120, 160mg/5 ml; 500mg/15ml; drops 80mg/0.8ml & 80mg/1.66ml, & 100mg/ml; supp 80, 120, 125, 300, 325, & 650mg] ▸LK ♀B ▸+ $

tramadol (*Ultram*): Moderate to moderately severe pain: 50-100mg tab(s) PO q4-6h prn, max 400mg/day. Adjust dose in elderly, renal & hepatic dysfunction. Avoid in opioid dependent patients. Seizures may occur with concurrent antidepressants. [Trade: Tabs immediate release (q4-6h) 50mg.] ▸KL ♀C ▸- $$$$

ANESTHESIA

Anesthetics & Sedatives

etomidate (*Amidate*): Induction 0.3 mg/kg IV. ▸L ♀C ▸? $

fentanyl (*Sublimaze, Oralet*): IV adjunct to general anesthesia & procedural sedation, specialized dosing. [Trade: Oralet lozenges 100,200,300,400 mcg] ▸L ♀C ▸? ©II $

ketamine (*Ketalar*): 1-2 mg/kg IV over 1-2 min or 4 mg/kg IM induces 10-20 min dissociative state. Concurrent atropine minimizes hypersalivation. ▸L ♀? ▸? $

methohexital (*Brevital*): Induction 1-1.5 mg/kg IV, duration 5 min. ▸L ♀B ▸? ©IV $

midazolam (*Versed*): Adult sedation/anxiolysis: 5 mg or 0.07 mg/kg IM; or 1 mg IV slowly q2-3 min up to 5 mg. Peds: 0.25-1.0 mg/kg to max of 20 mg PO, or 0.1-0.15 mg/kg IM. IV route (6 mo to 5 yo): Initial dose 0.05-0.1 mg/kg IV, then titrated to max 0.6 mg/kg. IV route (6-12 yo): Initial dose 0.025-0.05 mg/kg IV, then titrated to max 0.4 mg/kg. Monitor for resp depression. [Oral liquid 2 mg/ml] ▸LK ♀D ▸- ©IV $

propofol (*Diprivan*): 40 mg IV q10 sec until induction (2-2.5 mg/kg) ICU ventilator sedation: infusion 5-50 mcg/kg/min. ▸L ♀B ▸- $$$

thiopental (*Pentothal*): Induction 3-5 mg/kg IV, duration 5 min. ▸L ♀C ▸? ©III $

Local Anesthetics

bupivacaine (*Marcaine, Sensorcaine*): 0.25% injection. [0.25%. With epinephrine: 0.25%] ▸LK ♀C ▸? $

etidocaine (*Duranest*): 1% injection. [1% solution. With epi: 1%, 1.5%.] ▸LK ♀B ▸? $

lidocaine (*Xylocaine*): 0.5-1% injection with and without epinephrine. [0.5,1,1.5,2%. With epi: 0.5,1,1.5,2%.] ▸LK ♀B ▸? $

mepivacaine (*Carbocaine*): 1-2% injection. [1,1.5,2,3%.] ▸LK ♀C ▸? $

Neuromuscular Blockers

cisatracurium (*Nimbex*): 0.1-0.2 mg/kg IV. Duration 30-60 min. ▸Plasma ♀B ▸? $$

mivacurium (*Mivacron*): 0.15 mg/kg IV. Duration 20 minutes. ▸Plasma ♀C ▸? $

pancuronium (*Pavulon*): 0.04 to 0.1 mg/kg IV. Duration 45 min. ▸LK ♀C ▸? $

rapacuronium (*Raplon*): Tracheal intubation (adult): 1.5 mg/kg IV. Repeat dosing 0.5 mg/kg IV as needed. Tracheal intubation (child), 2 mg/kg IV. ▸KL ♀C ▸? $

rocuronium (*Zemuron*): 0.6 mg/kg IV. Duration 30 min. ▶L ♀B ▶? $$
succinylcholine (*Anectine, Quelicin*): 0.6-1.1 mg/kg IV. Peds: 2 mg/kg IV, preceded by atropine 0.02 mg/kg if <5 yo. ▶Plasma ♀C ▶? $
vecuronium (*Norcuron*): 0.08-0.1 mg/kg IV. Duration 15-30 min. ▶LK ♀C ▶? $

ANTIMICROBIALS

Aminoglycosides (see also dermatology, ophthalmology, & peds dosing table)
amikacin (*Amikin*): 15 mg/kg up to 1500 mg/day IM/IV divided q8-12h. Peak 20-35 mcg/ml, trough <5 mcg/ml. Alternative 15mg/kg IV q24h. ▶K ♀D ▶? $$$$
gentamicin (*Garamycin, Cidomycin*): Adults: 3-5 mg/kg/day IM/IV divided q8h. Peak 5-10 mcg/ml, trough <2 mcg/ml. Alternative 5-7 mg/kg IV q24h. Children: 2-2.5 mg/kg q8h. ▶K ♀D ▶? $$
tobramycin (*Nebcin, TOBI*): Adults: 3-5 mg/kg/day IM/IV divided q8h. Peak 5-10 mcg/ml, trough <2 mcg/ml. Alternative 5-7 mg/kg IV q24h. Children: 2-2.5 mg/kg q8h. Cystic fibrosis (TOBI): 300 mg neb bid 28 days on, then 28 days off. [TOBI 300 mg ampules for nebulizer.] ▶K ♀D ▶? $$$$

Antifungal Agents
amphotericin B deoxycholate (*Fungizone*): Test dose 0.1 mg/kg up to 1 mg slow IV. Wait 2-4 hours, and if tolerated then begin 0.25 mg/kg IV qd and advance to 0.5-1.5 mg/kg/day depending on fungal type. Maximum dose 1.5 mg/kg/day. Oral candidiasis: 1 ml oral susp swish & swallow qid given between meals x at least 2 weeks. [Trade: Oral susp 100 mg/ml.] ▶Tissues ♀B for IV, C for PO ▶? $$$
amphotericin B lipid formulations (*Amphotec, Abelcet, AmBisome*): Abelcet: 5 mg/kg/day IV at 2.5 mg/kg/hr. AmBisome: 3-5 mg/kg/day IV over 2 h. Amphotec. Test dose of 10 ml over 15-30 minutes, observe for 30 minutes, then 3-4 mg/kg/day IV at 1 mg/kg/hour. ▶? ♀B ▶? $$$$$
clotrimazole (*Mycelex*): Oral troches 5 times/day x 14 days. [Trade: Oral troches 10.] ▶L ♀C ▶? $$$
fluconazole (*Diflucan*): Oropharyngeal/esophageal candidiasis: 200 mg IV/PO first day, then 100 mg IV/PO qd. Vaginal candidiasis: 150 mg PO single dose. Systemic candidiasis, cryptococcal meningitis: 400 mg IV/PO qd. Peds: Oropharyngeal/esophageal candidiasis: 6 mg/kg IV/PO first day, then 3 mg/kg IV/PO qd. Systemic candidiasis: 6-12 mg/kg IV/PO qd. Cryptococcal meningitis: 12 mg/kg IV/PO on first day, then 6 mg/kg IV/PO qd. [Trade: Tabs 50,100,150,200, susp 10 & 40 mg/ml.] ▶K ♀C ▶- $$$$
flucytosine (*Ancobon*): 50-150 mg/kg/day PO divided qid. Myelosuppression. [Trade: Caps 250, 500.] ▶K ♀C ▶- $$$$$
griseofulvin microsize (*Fulvicin-U/F, Grifulvin-V*): Tinea: 11 mg/kg up to 500 mg PO qd x 4-6 weeks. [Generic/Trade: Tabs 500. Trade: Tabs 250, caps 250, susp 125 mg/5ml.] ▶Skin ♀C ▶? $$
itraconazole (*Sporanox*): Onychomycosis "pulse dosing": 200 mg PO bid for 1st wk of month x 2 months (fingernails) or 3-4 months (toenails). Oral sol'n for oropharyngeal or esophageal candidiasis: 100-200 mg qd or 100 mg bid swish & swallow in 10 ml increments on empty stomach. For life-threatening infections, load with 200 mg IV bid x 4 doses or 200 mg PO tid x 3 days. Contraindicated with cisapride, lovastatin, PO midazolam, pimozide, quinidine, simvastatin, triazolam. [Trade: Cap 100, oral sol'n 10 mg/ml.] ▶L ♀C ▶- $$$$$

ketoconazole (*Nizoral*): 200-400 mg PO qd. Hepatotoxicity. Contraindicated with cisapride, midazolam, pimozide, triazolam. H2 blockers, proton pump inhibitors, antacids impair absorption. [Generic/Trade: Tabs 200.] ▶L ♀C ▶- $$$$

nystatin (*Mycostatin, Nadostine, Nilstat, Nyaderm*): Thrush: 4-6 ml PO swish & swallow qid. Infants: 2 ml/dose with 1 ml in each cheek qid. [Generic/Trade: Susp 100,000 units/ml. Trade: Troches 200,000 units.] ▶Not absorbed ♀B ▶? $

terbinafine (*Lamisil*): Onychomycosis: 250 mg PO qd x 6 weeks for fingernails, x 12 weeks for toenails. "Pulse dosing": 500 mg PO qd for first week of month x 2 months (fingernails) or 4 months (toenails). [Trade: Tabs 250.] ▶LK ♀B ▶- $$$$$

Antimalarials

chloroquine phosphate (*Aralen*): Malaria prophylaxis for chloroquine sensitive areas: 8 mg/kg up to 500 mg PO q wk from 1-2 wks before exposure to 4 wks post exposure. [Trade: Tabs 250,500 (500 mg phosphate equiv to 300 base).] ▶KL ♀C but + ▶+ $

doxycycline (*Vibramycin, Vibra-Tabs, Doryx, Doxycin*): Malaria prophylaxis: 2 mg/kg/day up to 100 mg PO qd starting 1-2 days before exposure until 4 weeks after. 100 mg IV/PO bid for severe infections. [Generic/Trade: Tabs 100, caps 50,100. Trade: Susp 25 mg/5 ml, syrup 50 mg/5ml (contains sulfites).] ▶LK ♀D ▶? $

Malarone (atovaquone and proguanil): Prevention of malaria: 1 adult tab PO qd from 1-2 days before exposure until 7 days after. Treatment of malaria: 4 adult tabs PO qd x 3 days. Take with food or milky drink. [Trade: Adult tabs atovaquone 250/proguanil 100; pediatric tabs atovaquone 62.5/proguanil 25.] ▶Fecal excretion; LK ♀C ▶? ?

mefloquine (*Lariam*): Malaria prophylaxis for chloroquine-resistant areas: 250 mg PO q week from 1 week before exposure to 4 weeks after. Treatment: 1250 mg PO single dose. [Trade: Tabs 250.] ▶L ♀C ▶? $$

primaquine phosphate: 26.3 mg PO qd x 14 days. [Generic: Tabs 26.3 (equiv to 15 mg base).] ▶L ♀- ▶- $

Antimyocobacterial Agents

dapsone (*Avlosulfon*): Pneumocystis prophylaxis, leprosy: 100 mg PO qd. Pneumocystis treatment: 100 mg PO qd with trimethoprim 5 mg/kg PO tid x 21 days. [Generic: Tabs 25,100.] ▶LK ♀C ▶+? $

ethambutol (*Myambutol, Etibi*): 15-25 mg/kg up to 2500 mg PO qd. [Trade: Tabs 100, 400.] ▶LK ♀B ▶+ $$$$$

ethionamide (*Trecator-SC*): 15-20 mg/kg/day up to 1 g PO divided bid. [Trade: Tabs 250.] ▶L ♀- ▶? $$$$$

isoniazid (*INH, Isotamine*): 10-20 mg/kg up to 300 mg PO qd. Hepatotoxicity. Consider supplemental pyridoxine 10-25 mg PO qd. [Generic: Tabs 100,300, syrup 50 mg/5 ml.] ▶LK ♀C but + ▶+ $

pyrazinamide (*Tebrazid*): 15-30 mg/kg up to 2000 mg PO qd. [Generic: Tabs 500.] ▶LK ♀C ▶? $$$

rifabutin (*Mycobutin*): 300 mg PO qd or 150 mg PO bid. [Trade: Caps 150.] ▶L ♀B ▶? $$$$$

Rifamate (isoniazid + rifampin): 2 caps PO qd. [Trade: Caps isoniazid 150 + rifampin 300.] ▶LK ♀C ▶+ $$$$

rifampin (*Rimactane, Rifadin, Rofact*): 10-20 mg/kg up to 600 mg PO/IV qd. [Generic/Trade: Caps 150,300. Pharmacists can make oral susp.] ▶L ♀C ▶+ $$$

rifapentine (*Priftin*): 600 mg PO twice weekly x 2 months, then once weekly x 4 months (twice weekly if HIV). [Trade: Tabs 150.] ▶Esterases, then fecal ♀C ▶? $$$

Rifater (isoniazid + rifampin + pyrazinamide): 6 tabs PO qd if weight 55+ kg, 5 tabs per day if 45-54 kg, 4 per day if ≤44 kg. [Trade: Tab Isoniazid 50 + rifampin 120 + pyrazinamide 300 mg.] ▶LK ♀C ▶? $$$$$

Antiparasitics

albendazole (*Albenza*): Hydatid disease or neurocysticercosis: 400 mg PO bid, duration varies. If <60 kg, then 15 mg/kg/d, max 800 mg/d. [Trade: Tabs 200.] ▶L ♀C ▶? $$$

atovaquone (*Mepron*): Pneumocystis treatment: 750 mg PO bid x 21 days. Pneumocystis prevention: 1500 mg PO qd. Take with meals. [Trade: Susp 750 mg/5 ml, foil pouch 750 mg/5ml, 1500 mg/10 ml.] ▶Fecal excretion ♀C ▶? $$$$$

ivermectin (*Stromectol*): Single PO dose of 200 mcg/kg for strongyloidiasis, scabies (not children <15 kg), 150 mcg/kg for onchocerciasis. [Trade: Tab 6 mg.] ▶L ♀C ▶? $

mebendazole (*Vermox*): Pinworm: 100 mg PO single dose; consider repeat dose in 2 wks. Roundworm, whipworm, hookworm: 100 mg PO bid x 3d. [Trade/Generic: Chew tab 100.] ▶L ♀C ▶? $

metronidazole (*Flagyl, Trikacide*): Trichomoniasis: 2g PO single dose for patient & sex partners. Giardia: 250 mg PO tid x 5-7 days. [Generic/Trade: Tabs 250,500. Trade: Caps 375, Flagyl ER tabs 750.] ▶KL ♀B(- in 1st trimester) ▶?- $

pentamidine (*Pentam, NebuPent, Pentacarinat*): Pneumocystis treatment: 4 mg/kg IM/IV qd x 14-21 days. Pneumocystis prevention: 300 mg nebulized q 4 weeks. [Trade: Aerosol 300.] ▶K ♀C ▶- $$$$$

pyrantel (*Pin-X, Pinworm, Combantrin*): Pinworm and roundworm: 11 mg/kg up to 1g PO single dose. [OTC: Caps 62.5 mg, liquid 50 mg/ml.] ▶Not absorbed ♀- ▶? $

pyrimethamine (*Daraprim*): Toxoplasmosis: 50-75 mg PO qd x 1-3 weeks, then reduce dose by 50% for 4-5 more weeks. CNS toxoplasmosis in AIDS: 200 mg PO x 1, then 75-100 mg qd. Secondary prevention after CNS toxoplasmosis in AIDS: 25-75 mg PO qd. Peds: 1 mg/kg/day PO divided bid x 2-4 days, then reduce by 50% x 1 month. [Trade: Tabs 25.] ▶L ♀C ▶- $$

Antiviral Agents - Anti-CMV

cidofovir (*Vistide*): CMV retinitis in AIDS: Induction 5 mg/kg IV q week x 2 wks, maintenance 5 mg/kg every other week. Nephrotoxicity. ▶K ♀C ▶- $$$$$

foscarnet (*Foscavir*): CMV retinitis: Induction 60 mg/kg IV q8h x 2-3 weeks, each dose over 1h. Maintenance 90-120 mg/kg/day IV over 2h. HSV infections: 40 mg/kg q8-12h, each dose over 1h. Nephrotoxicity, seizures. ▶K ♀C ▶? $$$$$

ganciclovir (*DHPG, Cytovene*): CMV retinitis: Induction 5 mg/kg IV q12h for 14-21 days. Maintenance 6 mg/kg IV qd for 5 days per week. Oral: 1000 mg PO tid or 500 mg 6 times daily. [Trade: Caps 250, 500.] ▶K ♀C ▶- $$$$$

Antiviral Agents - Anti-Herpetic

acyclovir (*Zovirax, Avirax*): 5-10 mg/kg IV q8h, each dose over 1h. Genital herpes: 400 mg PO tid x 7-10 days for first episode, x 5 days for recurrent episodes. Herpes prophylaxis: 400 mg PO bid. Zoster: 800 mg PO 5 times/day x 7-10 days. Varicella: 20 mg/kg up to 800 mg PO qid x 5 days. [Generic/Trade: Caps 200, tabs 400,800 Trade: Susp 200 mg/5 ml.] ▶K ♀B ▶+ $$

famciclovir (*Famvir*): First-episode genital herpes: 250 mg PO tid x 7-10 days. Recurrent genital herpes: 125 mg PO bid x 5 days. Herpes prophylaxis: 250 mg PO bid. Recurrent oral/genital herpes in HIV patients: 500 bid x 7 days. Zoster: 500 mg PO tid for 7 days. [Trade: Tabs 125,250,500.] ▶K ♀B ▶? $$$

valacyclovir (*Valtrex*): First episode genital herpes: 1000 mg PO bid x 10 days. Recurrent genital herpes: 500 mg PO bid x 5 days. Herpes prophylaxis: 500-1000 mg PO qd. Zoster: 1000 mg PO tid x 7 days. [Trade: Tabs 500,1000.] ▶K ♀B ▶? $$$

Antiviral Agents - Anti-HIV - Non-Nucleoside Reverse Transcriptase Inhibitors (Many serious drug interactions - always check before prescribing!)

delavirdine (*Rescriptor*): Adults & children >16yo: 400 mg PO tid. [Trade: Tabs 100,200.] ▶L ♀C ▶- $$$$$

efavirenz (*Sustiva*): Adults & children >40kg: 600 mg PO qhs. [Trade: Caps 50,100,200.] ▶L ♀C ▶- $$$$$

nevirapine (*Viramune*): 200 mg PO qd x 14 days initially. If tolerated, increase to 200 mg PO bid. Occasional severe skin reactions & hepatotoxicity. [Trade: Tabs 200, susp 50mg/5ml.] ▶LK ♀C ▶- $$$$$

Antiviral Agents - Anti-HIV - Nucleoside Reverse Transcriptase Inhibitors

abacavir (*Ziagen*): Adult: 300 mg PO bid. Children >3 mo: 8 mg/kg PO bid up to 300 mg PO bid. Potentially fatal hypersensitivity reactions (Never rechallenge if this occurs), lactic acidosis with hepatic steatosis. [Trade: Tabs 300, oral sol'n 20 mg/ml.] ▶L ♀C ▶- $$$$$

Combivir (lamivudine+zidovudine): 1 tab PO bid. [Trade: Tabs lamivudine 150 + zidovudine 300.] ▶LK ♀C ▶- $$$$$

didanosine (*Videx, ddI*): Adult >60 kg: 400 mg PO qd or 200 mg PO bid. Adult <60 kg: 250 mg PO qd or 125 mg PO bid. Peds: 120 mg/m2 PO bid. [Trade: Chewable/dispersible buffered tabs 25,50,100,150,200, packets of buffered powder for oral sol'n 100,167,250, pediatric powder for oral sol'n 10 mg/ml.] ▶LK ♀B ▶- $$$$$

lamivudine (*Epivir, Epivir-HBV, 3TC, Heptovir*): Epivir for HIV infection. Adults: 2 mg/kg up to 150 mg PO bid. Peds: 4mg/kg up to 150 mg PO bid. Epivir-HBV for hepatitis B: Adults: 100 mg PO qd [Trade: Epivir, 3TC: Tabs 150, oral sol'n 10 mg/ml. Epivir-HBV, Heptovir. Tabs 100, oral sol'n 5 mg/ml.] ▶K ♀C ▶- $$$$$

stavudine (*Zerit, d4T*): 40 mg PO q12h, or 30 mg q12h if <60 kg. Peds (<30 kg): 1 mg/kg PO bid. [Trade: Caps 15,20,30,40; oral sol'n 1 mg/ml.] ▶LK ♀C ▶- $$$$$

zalcitabine (*Hivid, ddC*): 0.75 mg PO q8h. [Trade: Tabs 0.375,0.75.] ▶K ♀C ▶- $$$$$

zidovudine (*Retrovir, AZT, azidothymidine, ZDV*): 200mg PO tid or 300 bid. Peds: 180mg/m^2 up to 200 mg q6h. [Trade: Cap 100, tab 300, syrup 50 mg/5ml.] ▶LK ♀C ▶- $$$$$

Antiviral Agents - Anti-HIV - Protease Inhibitors

NOTE: Many serious drug interactions - always check before prescribing!

amprenavir (*Agenerase*): 1200 mg PO bid. Peds >4yo: caps 20 mg/kg PO bid up to 1200 mg bid. Oral sol'n 22.5 mg/kg PO bid up to 2800 mg/day. [Trade: Caps 50,150, oral sol'n 15mg/ml.] ▶L ♀C ▶- $$$$$

indinavir (*Crixivan*): 800 mg PO q8h between meals with water (at least 48 ounces per day to prevent kidney stones). [Trade: Caps 200,333,400.] ▶LK ♀C ▶- $$$$$

nelfinavir (*Viracept*): 750 mg PO tid or 1250 mg PO bid with meals. [Trade: Tab 250, powder 50 mg/g.] ▶L ♀B ◗- $$$$$

ritonavir (*Norvir*): Begin 300 mg PO bid with meals, and increase over 1-2 weeks to 600 mg bid. [Trade: Cap 100, oral sol'n 80 mg/ml.] ▶L ♀B ◗- $$$$$

saquinavir (*Fortovase, Invirase*): Fortovase: 1200 mg PO tid. Invirase: 600 mg PO tid. Fortovase preferred over Invirase. Take with/after meals. [Trade: Fortovase (soft gel), Invirase (hard gel) caps 200.] ▶L ♀B ◗? $$$$$

Antiviral Agents - Anti-Influenza

amantadine (*Symmetrel*): Influenza A: 100 mg PO bid. Elderly: 100 mg qd. Peds: 5 mg/kg up to 150 mg/day. [Generic: Cap 100. Trade: Tab 100. Generic/Trade: Syrup 50mg/5ml.] ▶K ♀C ◗? $

oseltamivir (*Tamiflu*): 75 mg PO bid x 5 days starting within 2 days of symptom onset. [Trade: Caps 75.] ▶Esterases, then K ♀C ◗? $$$

rimantadine (*Flumadine*): Influenza A: 100 mg PO bid x 7 days. Peds: 5 mg/kg PO qd up to 150 mg/day. [Trade: Tabs 100, syrup 50 mg/5 ml.] ▶LK ♀C ◗- $

zanamivir (*Relenza*): Influenza treatment: 2 puffs bid x 5 days. [Trade: Rotadisk inhaler 5 mg/puff (20 puffs).] ▶K ♀C ◗? $$

Carbapenems

imipenem-cilastatin (*Primaxin*): 250-1000 mg IV q6-8h. ▶K ♀C ◗? $$$$$

meropenem (*Merrem IV*): 1 g IV q8h. Peds: 20-40 mg/kg up to 2g/dose IV q8h. ▶K ♀B ◗? $$$$$

Cephalosporins - 1st Generation

cefadroxil (*Duricef*): 1-2 g/day PO divided qd/bid. Peds: 30 mg/kg/day divided bid. [Generic/Trade: Tabs 1000, caps 500. Trade: Susp 125,250,500 mg/5ml.] ▶K ♀B ◗+ $$$

cefazolin (*Ancef, Kefzol*): 0.5-1.5 g IM/IV q6-8h. Peds: 25-50 mg/kg/day divided q6-8h, severe infections 100 mg/kg/day. ▶K ♀B ◗+ $$$

cephalexin (*Keflex, Keftab*): 250-500 mg PO qid. Peds 25-50 mg/kg/day. Not for otitis media and sinusitis. [Generic/Trade: Caps 250,500, tabs 250,500, susp 125 & 250 mg/5ml. Keftab: 500.] ▶K ♀B ◗? $

Cephalosporins - 2nd Generation

cefaclor (*Ceclor*): 250-500 mg PO tid. Peds: 20-40 mg/kg/day PO divided bid for otitis media & pharyngitis, or tid for other infections. Extended release (Ceclor CD): 375-500 mg PO bid. Serum sickness-like reactions can occur with repeated use. [Generic/Trade: Caps 250,500, susp 125,187,250,375 mg/5ml; Extended release (Ceclor CD) 375,500.] ▶K ♀B ◗? $$$

cefotetan (*Cefotan*): 1-2 g IM/IV q12h. ▶K/Bile ♀B ◗? $$$$$

cefoxitin (*Mefoxin*): 1-2 g IM/IV q6-8h. ▶K ♀B ◗+ $$$$$

cefprozil (*Cefzil*): 250-500 mg PO qd or divided bid. Pediatric otitis media: 15 mg/kg/dose PO bid. Peds pharyngitis: 7.5 mg/kg/dose PO bid x 10d. [Trade: Tabs 250,500, susp 125 & 250 mg/5ml.] ▶K ♀B ◗+ $$$

cefuroxime (*Zinacef, Ceftin, Kefurox*): 750-1500 mg IM/IV q8h. Peds: 50-100 mg/kg/day IV divided q6-8h, not for meningitis. 250-500 mg PO bid. Peds: 20-30 mg/kg/d susp PO divided bid. [Trade: Tabs 125,250,500, susp 125 & 250mg/5ml.] ▶K ♀B ◗? $$$

loracarbef (*Lorabid*): 200-400 mg PO bid. Peds: 30 mg/kg/day for otitis media (15 mg/kg/day for other infections) divided bid. [Trade. Caps 200,400, susp 100 & 200 mg/5ml.] ▶K ♀B ▶? $$$

Cephalosporins - 3rd Generation

cefdinir (*Omnicef*): 600 mg PO qd or 300 mg PO bid. Peds: 14 mg/kg/day divided qd/bid. [Trade: Cap 300, susp 125 mg/5ml.] ▶K ♀B ▶? $$$

cefixime (*Suprax*): 400 mg PO qd or 200 bid. Gonorrhea: 400 mg PO single-dose. Peds: 8 mg/kg/day divided qd/bid. [Trade: Tabs 200,400, susp 100 mg/5 ml.] ▶K/Bile ♀B ▶? $$$

cefoperazone (*Cefobid*): Usual dose 2-4 g/day IM/IV given q12h. Maximum dose: 6-12 g/day IV given q6-12 h. Possible clotting impairment. ▶Bile/K ♀B ▶? $$$$$

cefotaxime (*Claforan*): Usual dose: 1-2 g IM/IV q6-8h. Peds: 50-180 mg/kg/day IM/IV divided q4-6h. Use high end of dosage range for meningitis. ▶KL ♀B ▶+ $$$$$

cefpodoxime (*Vantin*): 100-400 mg PO bid. Peds: 10 mg/kg/d divided bid for pharyngitis; or qd for otitis. [Trade: Tabs 100,200, susp 50 & 100 mg/5ml.] ▶K ♀B ▶? $$$

ceftazidime (*Ceptaz, Fortaz, Tazidime, Tazicef*): 1 g IM/IV or 2 g IV q8-12h. Peds: 30-50 mg/kg IV q8h. ▶K ♀B ▶+ $$$$$

ceftibuten (*Cedax*): 400 mg PO qd. Peds: 9 mg/kg up to 400 mg PO qd. [Trade: Cap 400, susp 90 & 180 mg/5 ml.] ▶K ♀B ▶? $$$

ceftizoxime (*Cefizox*): 1-2 g IV q8-12h. Peds: 50 mg/kg/dose IV q6-8h. ▶K ♀B ▶? $$$$$

ceftriaxone (*Rocephin*): 1-2 g IM/IV q24h. Meningitis: 2 g IV q12h. Gonorrhea: single dose 125 mg IM (250 if treating PID). Peds: 50-75 mg/kg/day (max 2g) divided q12-24h. 100 mg/kg/day (max 4g) for meningitis. Pediatric acute otitis media: 50 mg/kg up to 1000 mg IM single dose. Dilute in 1% lidocaine for IM use. ▶K/Bile ♀B ▶+ $$$$$

SEXUALLY TRANSMITTED DISEASES & VAGINITIS *MMWR 1998; 47*

Bacterial vaginosis: 1) metronidazole 5 g of 0.75% gel intravaginally bid or qhs for 5 days 2) clindamycin 5 g of 2% cream intravaginally qhs for 7 days. 3) metronidazole 500 mg PO bid for 7 days or extended-release 750 mg PO qd for 7 days. In pregnancy (2nd or 3rd trimesters): metronidazole 250 mg PO tid for 7 days.

Candidal vaginitis: 1) intravaginal clotrimazole, miconazole, terconazole, nystatin, tioconazole, or butoconazole. 2) fluconazole 150 mg PO single dose.

Chlamydia: 1) azithromycin 1 g PO single dose. 2) doxycycline 100 mg PO bid x 7d. 3) ofloxacin 300 mg PO bid x 7d. 4) erythromycin base 500 mg PO qid x 7d.

Gonorrhea: 1) ceftriaxone 125 mg IM single dose. 2) cefixime 400 mg PO single dose. 3) ciprofloxacin 500 mg PO single dose. 4) ofloxacin 400 mg PO single dose.

Herpes simplex (genital first episode): 1) acyclovir 400 mg PO tid for 7-10 days. 2) famciclovir 250 PO tid for 7-10 days. 3) valacyclovir 1 g PO bid for 7-10 days.

Herpes simplex (genital, recurrent): 1) acyclovir 400 mg PO tid for 5 days. 2) famciclovir 125 mg PO bid for 5 days. 3) valacyclovir 500 mg PO bid for 5 days.

Herpes simplex (suppressive therapy): 1) acyclovir 400mg PO bid. 2) famciclovir 250 mg PO bid. 3) valacyclovir 250 mg PO bid or 500-1000 mg PO qd.

Pelvic inflammatory disease (PID), outpatient treatment: 1) ceftriaxone 250 mg IM + doxycycline 100 mg PO bid for 14 days. 2) ofloxacin 400 mg PO bid + metronidazole 500 mg PO bid for 14 days.

Trichomonal vaginitis: metronidazole 2 g PO single dose or 500 mg bid for 7days. Can use 2 g single dose in pregnant women. *See deluxe edition for unabbreviated table*

Cephalosporins - 4th Generation

cefepime (*Maxipime*): 0.5-2 g IM/IV q12h. ▶K ♀B ▶? $$$$$

Macrolides

azithromycin (*Zithromax*): 500 mg IV qd. Oral: 10 mg/kg up to 500 mg PO on 1st day, followed by 5 mg/kg up to 250 mg PO qd to complete 5 days. Pharyngitis: 12 mg/kg up to 500 mg PO qd x 5 days. Chlamydia, chancroid: 1g PO single dose. Mycobacterium avium complex prevention: 1200 mg PO q wk. [Trade: Tab 250,600, packet 1000, susp 100 & 200 mg/5 ml. Z-Pak: #6, 250 mg tabs.] ▶L ♀B ▶? $$

clarithromycin (*Biaxin, Biaxin XL*): 250-500 mg PO bid. Peds: 7.5 mg/kg PO bid. H pylori: See table in GI section. Mycobacterium avium complex prevention: 7.5 mg/kg up to 500 mg PO bid. Biaxin XL: 1000 mg PO qd with food. [Trade: Tab 250,500, susp 125 & 250 mg/5ml; Extended release (Biaxin XL) 500. Biaxin XL-Pak: #14, 500 mg tabs.] ▶KL ♀C ▶? $$$

erythromycin base (*Eryc, E-mycin*): 250-500 mg PO qid, 333 mg PO tid, or 500 mg PO bid. [Generic/Trade: Tab 250,333,500, cap delayed-release 250.] ▶L ♀B ▶+ $

erythromycin ethyl succinate (*EES*): 400 mg PO qid. Peds: 30-50 mg/kg/d divided qid. [Generic/Trade: Tab 400, susp 200&400 mg/5ml. Trade: Chew tab 200.] ▶L ♀B ▶+ $

erythromycin lactobionate (*Erythrocin*): 15-20 mg/kg/day (max 4g) IV divided q6h. Peds: 15-50 mg/kg/day IV divided q6h. ▶L ♀B ▶+ $$$$$

Pediazole (erythromycin ethyl succinate + sulfisoxazole): 50 mg/kg/day (based on EES dose) PO divided tid-qid. [Generic/Trade: Susp, erythromycin ethyl succinate 200 mg, sulfisoxazole 600 mg/5ml.] ▶KL ♀C ▶- $

Penicillins - 1st generation - Natural

benzathine penicillin (*Bicillin L-A*): 1.2 million units IM. Peds <27 kg 0.3-0.6 MU IM, ≥27 kg 0.9 MU IM. Doses last 2-4 wks. ▶K ♀B ▶? $

Bicillin CR (procaine and benzathine penicillin): combination of procaine and benzathine penicillin for IM use [Trade: for IM use in mixes of 1.2/1.2 million, 300/300, 600/600, 300/900 thousand units procaine/benzathine penicillin.] ▶K ♀B ▶? $

penicillin G: Pneumococcal pneumonia & severe infections: 250,000-400,000 units/kg/d (or 8-12 million units in an adult) IV divided q4-6h. Pneumococcal meningitis: 250,000 units/kg/day (or 24 million units in an adult) IV divided q2-4h. ▶K ♀B ▶? $$$

penicillin V (*Pen-Vee K, Veetids, Ledercillin VK*): Adults: 250-500 mg PO qid. AHA dosing for pharyngitis: 500 mg PO bid-tid x 10 days. Peds: 25-50 mg/kg/day divided bid-qid. AHA peds dosing for pharyngitis: 250 mg PO bid-tid x 10 days. [Generic/Trade: Tabs 250,500, oral sol'n 125 & 250 mg/5ml.] ▶K ♀B ▶? $

procaine penicillin (*Wycillin*): 0.6-1.2 million units IM (peak 4h, lasts 24h). ▶K ♀B ▶? $

Penicillins - 2nd generation - Penicillinase-Resistant

dicloxacillin (*Dynapen*): 125-500 mg PO qid. Peds: 12.5-25 mg/kg/day divided qid. [Generic/Trade: Caps 250,500. Trade: Susp 62.5 mg/5ml.] ▶KL ♀B ▶? $

nafcillin (*Nallpen*): 1-2 g IM/IV q4h. Peds: 50-200 mg/kg/day divided q4-6h. ▶L ♀B ▶? $$$$

oxacillin (*Bactocill*): 1-2 g IM/IV q4-6h. 500-1000 mg PO q4-6h. Peds 50-100 mg/kg/day PO divided qid. [Generic: Caps 250,500, oral sol'n 250 mg/5ml.] ▶KL ♀B ▶? $

Penicillins - 3rd generation - Aminopenicillins

amoxicillin (*Amoxil, Polymox, Trimox*): 250-500 mg PO tid, or 500-875 mg PO bid. Peds: 40 mg/kg/day PO divided tid or 45 mg/kg/day divided bid. Otitis media due to penicillin-resistant S pneumoniae: 80-90 mg/kg/day PO divided tid. Prevention of recurrent otitis media: 20 mg/kg PO qd. [Generic/Trade: Caps 250,500, chewables 125,250, susp 125, 250 mg/5ml. Trade: Tabs 500,875, chewables 200,400, susp 200 & 400mg/5ml, infant drops 50 mg/ml.] ▶K ♀B ◗+ $

amoxicillin clavulanate (*Augmentin, Clavulin*): 500-875 mg PO bid or 250-500 mg tid. Peds: 45 mg/kg/d PO divided bid or 40 mg/kg/d divided tid for otitis, sinusitis, pneumonia; 25 mg/kg/d divided bid or 20 mg/kg/d divided tid for less severe infections. Otitis media due to penicillin-resistant S pneumoniae: amoxicillin 80-90 mg/kg/day + clavulanate not more than 10 mg/kg/day x 10 days. Can use standard doses of Augmentin with additional amoxicillin. [Trade: Tabs (amoxicillin/clavulanate) 250/125,500/125,875/125, chewables 125/31.25,200/28.5,250/62.5,400/57, susp 125/31.25, 200/28.5, 250/62.5, & 400/57mg/5ml .] ▶K ♀B ◗? $$$

ampicillin (*Principen, Ampicin*): Pneumonia, soft tissue infections: 250-500 mg IM/IV/ PO q6h. Gastrointestinal infections, UTIs: 500 mg IM/IV/PO q6h. Sepsis, meningitis: 150-200 mg/kg/day IV divided q3-4h. Peds: 50-400 mg/kg/day IM/ IV divided q4-6h. [Generic/Trade: Caps 250,500, susp 125 & 250 mg/ 5ml.] ▶K ♀B ◗? $$$

ampicillin sulbactam (*Unasyn*): 1.5-3 g IM/IV q6h. ▶K ♀B ◗? $$$$$

Penicillins - 4th generation - Extended Spectrum

mezlocillin (*Mezlin*): 3-4 g IM/IV q4-6h. Peds: 50 mg/kg IV q4h. ▶KL ♀B ◗? $$$$$

piperacillin (*Pipracil*): 3-4 g IM/IV q4-6h. ▶K/Bile ♀B ◗? $$$$$

piperacillin tazobactam (*Zosyn, Tazocin*): 3.375 g IV q4-6h. ▶K ♀B ◗? $$$$$

ticarcillin (*Ticar*): 3-4 g IM/IV q4-6h. Peds: 200-300 mg/kg/day divided q4-6h. ▶K ♀B ◗+ $$$$$

ticarcillin clavulanate (*Timentin*): 3.1 g IV q4-6h. Peds: 50 mg/kg up to 3.1 g IV q4-6h. ▶K ♀B ◗? $$$$$

Quinolones - 1st Generation

nalidixic acid (*NegGram*): 1 g PO qid. [Trade: Tabs 0.25,0.5,1 g, susp 250 mg/5ml.] ▶KL ♀C ◗? $$$$$

Quinolones - 2nd Generation

ciprofloxacin (*Cipro*): 200-400 mg IV q12h. 250-750 mg PO bid. Gonorrhea: 250 mg PO single dose. Simple UTI: 100 mg bid x 3d. [Trade: Tabs 100,250,500,750, susp 250 & 500 mg/5ml.] ▶LK ♀C ◗? $$$

enoxacin (*Penetrex*): 200-400 mg PO bid. [Trade: Tabs 200,400.] ▶LK ♀C ◗? $$

lomefloxacin (*Maxaquin*): 400 mg PO qd. Photosensitivity. [Trade: Tabs 400.] ▶LK ♀C ◗? $$$

norfloxacin (*Noroxin*): Simple UTI: 400 mg PO bid x 3 days. [Generic: Tabs 400.] ▶LK ♀C ◗? $$

ofloxacin (*Floxin*): 200-400 mg IV/PO q12h. [Trade tabs 200,300,400.] ▶LK ♀C ◗? $$$

Quinolones - 3rd Generation

levofloxacin (*Levaquin*): 250-500 mg PO/IV qd. [Trade: Tabs 250,500.] ▶KL ♀C ◗? $$$

sparfloxacin (*Zagam*): 400 mg PO first day, then 200 PO qd. [Trade: Tabs 200.] ▶KL ♀C ◗? $$$

Quinolones - 4th Generation

gatifloxacin (*Tequin*): 400 mg IV/PO qd. Simple UTI: 400 mg PO single dose or 200 mg PO qd x3d. Gonorrhea: 400 mg PO single dose. [Trade tabs 200,400.] ▶K ♀C ◗- $$$

moxifloxacin (*Avelox*): 400 mg PO qd. [Trade: Tabs 400.] ▶LK ♀C ◗- $$$

trovafloxacin (*Trovan*, alatrofloxacin): 200-300 mg IV q24h then 200 mg PO qd for not more than 14 days. Hepatotoxicity. Only for inpatient treatment of serious or life-threatening infections. [Trade: Tabs 100, 200.] ▶LK ♀C ◗- $$$

Sulfonamides

Bactrim, Cotrim, Septra, Sulfatrim (trimethoprim/sulfamethoxazole, TMP/SMX, cotrimoxazole): One tab PO bid, double strength (DS, 160/800) or single strength (80/400). Pneumocystis treatment: 15-20 mg/kg/day (based on TMP) IV divided q6-8h or PO divided q6h x 21 days total. Pneumocystis prophylaxis: 1 DS tab PO qd. Peds: 5 ml susp per 10 kg (up to 20 ml) per dose PO bid. [Generic/Trade: Tabs 80 TMP/400 SMX (single strength), 160 TMP/800 SMX (double strength; DS), susp 40 TMP/200 SMX per 5ml. 20 ml susp = 2 SS tabs = 1 DS tab.] ▶K ♀C ◗+ $

Pediazole (erythromycin ethyl succinate + sulfisoxazole): 50 mg/kg/day (based on EES dose) PO divided tid-qid. [Generic/Trade: Susp, erythromycin ethyl succinate 200 mg, sulfisoxazole 600 mg/5ml.] ▶KL ♀C ◗- $

sulfadiazine: Toxoplasmosis: 100-200 mg/kg/day PO up to 1-1.5 g qid with pyrimethamine and leucovorin. [Generic: Tab 500.] ▶K ♀C ◗+ $$$$$

sulfamethoxazole (*Gantanol*): 1000 mg PO bid. [Trade: Tabs 500.] ▶K ♀C ◗- $

sulfisoxazole (*Gantrisin Pediatric, Sulfizole*): Peds prophylaxis for recurrent otitis media: 50 mg/kg PO qhs. [Trade: susp 500 mg/5ml.] ▶KL ♀C ◗+ $

Tetracyclines

doxycycline (*Vibramycin, Doryx, Periostat, Doxycin*): 100 mg PO bid on first day, then 50 mg bid or 100 mg qd. 100 mg PO/IV bid for severe infections. Periostat for periodontitis: 20 mg PO bid. [Generic/Trade: Tabs 100, caps 50,100. Trade: Susp 25 mg/5 ml, syrup 50 mg/5ml (contains sulfites), Periostat: Caps 20.] ▶LK ♀D ◗? $

minocycline (*Minocin, Dynacin*): 200 mg IV/PO initially, then 100 mg q12h. [Generic/Trade: Caps 50,75,100. Trade: Susp 50 mg/5ml.] ▶LK ♀D ◗? $$

tetracycline (*Sumycin, Tetracyn*): 250-500 mg PO qid. [Generic/Trade: Caps 250,500. Trade: Tabs 250,500, susp 125 mg/ 5ml.] ▶LK ♀D ◗? $

Other Antimicrobials

aztreonam (*Azactam*): 0.5-2 g IM/IV q6-12h. Peds: 30 mg/kg q6-8h. ▶K ♀B ◗+ $$$$$

chloramphenicol (*Chloromycetin*): 50-100 mg/kg/day IV divided q6h. Aplastic anemia. ▶LK ♀C ◗- $$$$$

clindamycin (*Cleocin, Dalacin C*): 600-900 mg IV q8h. Each IM injection should be ≤600 mg. 150-450 mg PO qid. Peds: 20-40 mg/kg/day IV divided q6-8h or 8-25 mg/kg/day susp PO divided tid/qid. [Generic/Trade: Cap 150. Trade: Cap 75,300, oral sol'n 75 mg/5ml.] ▶L ♀B ◗? $$

fosfomycin (*Monurol*): Simple UTI: 3 g packet PO single-dose. [Trade: 3g] ▶K ♀B ◗? $$

linezolid (*Zyvox*): 400-600 mg IV/PO q12 h. Infuse over 30-120 minutes. Thrombocytopenia. MAO inhibitor. [Trade: Tabs 600, susp 100 mg/5 ml. 400 mg tab FDA-approved, but not marketed.] ▶Esterase, fecal excretion ♀C ▶? $$$$$

metronidazole (*Flagyl, Trikacide*): Bacterial vaginosis: 500 mg PO bid x 7 days or Flagyl ER 750 mg PO qd x 7 days. H pylori: See table in GI section. Anaerobic bacterial infections. Load 1 g or 15 mg/kg IV, then 500 mg or 7.5 mg/kg IV/PO q6h, each IV dose over 1h (not to exceed 4 g/day). [Generic/Trade: Tabs 250,500. Trade: Caps 375. Flagyl ER tabs 750.] ▶KL ♀B(- in 1st trimester) ▶?- $

nitrofurantoin (*Furadantin, Macrodantin, Macrobid*): 50-100 mg PO qid. Peds: 5-7 mg/kg/day divided qid. Sustained release: 100 mg PO bid. [Macrodantin: Caps 25,50,100, Furadantin: Susp 25 mg/5ml; Macrobid: Caps 100. Generic: Caps 50,100.] ▶KL ♀B ▶+? $$

rifampin (*Rimactane, Rifadin, Rofact*): 10-20 mg/kg up to 600 mg PO/IV qd. [Generic/Trade: Caps 150,300. Pharmacists can make oral susp.] ▶L ♀C ▶+ $$$

Synercid (quinupristin and dalfopristin): 7.5 mg/kg IV q8-12 h, each dose over 1 h. Not active against E. faecalis. ▶Bile ♀B ▶? $$$$$

trimethoprim (*Primsol, Proloprim*): 100 mg PO bid or 200 mg PO qd. [Generic/Trade: Tabs 100,200. Primsol: Oral sol'n 50 mg/5ml.] ▶K ♀C ▶- $

vancomycin (*Vancocin*): 1g IV q12h, each dose over 1h. Peds: 10-15 mg/kg IV q6h. Clostridium difficile diarrhea: 40 mg/kg up to 2000 mg/day PO divided tid/qid x 7 10 days. [Generic/Trade: oral sol'n 1 g/20 ml bottle. Trade: Caps 125,250, oral sol'n 500 mg/6 ml.] ▶K ♀C ▶? $$$$$

CARDIOVASCULAR

ACE Inhibitors

benazepril (*Lotensin*): HTN: Start 10 mg PO qd, max 80 mg/day. [Trade: Tabs, non-scored 5,10,20,40.] ▶LK ♀C (1st trimester) D (2nd & 3rd) ▶? $$

captopril (*Capoten*): HTN: Start 25 mg PO bid/tid, max 450 mg/day (max 150 mg/day typical). CHF: Start 6.25-12.5 mg PO bid/tid, usual dose 50-100 mg PO tid. [Generic/Trade: Tabs, scored 12.5,25,50,100.] ▶LK ♀C (1st trimester) D (2nd & 3rd) ▶+ $$$

enalapril (*Vasotec*): HTN: Start 5 mg/day PO qd or divided bid, max 40 mg/day. CHF: Start 2.5 mg PO bid, usual dose 10-20 mg PO bid. [Generic/Trade: Tabs, scored 2.5,5, non-scored 10, 20.] ▶LK ♀C (1st trimester) D (2nd & 3rd) ▶+ $$

fosinopril (*Monopril*): HTN: Start 10 mg PO qd, max 80 mg/day. CHF: Start 10 mg PO qd, usual dose 20-40 mg PO qd. [Trade: Tabs, scored 10, non-scored 20,40.] ▶L ♀C (1st trimester) D (2nd & 3rd) ▶? $$

lisinopril (*Prinivil, Zestril*): HTN: Start 10 mg PO qd, max 80 mg/day. CHF, acute MI: Start 2.5-5 mg PO qd, usual dose 5-20 mg PO qd, max dose 40 mg. [Trade: Tabs, non-scored 2.5,10,20,40, scored 5.] ▶K ♀C (1st trimester) D (2nd & 3rd) ▶? $$

moexipril (*Univasc*): HTN: Start 7.5 mg PO qd, max 30 mg/day qd or divided bid. [Trade: Tabs, scored 7.5,15.] ▶LK ♀C (1st trimester) D (2nd & 3rd) ▶? $

perindopril (*Aceon*): HTN: Start 4 mg PO qd, max 16 mg/day. [Trade: Tabs, scored 2,4,8.] ▶K ♀C (1st trimester) D (2nd & 3rd) ▶? $$

quinapril (*Accupril*): HTN: Start 10 mg PO qd or divided bid, max 80 mg/day, CHF: Start 5 mg PO bid, usual dose 20 mg bid. [Trade: Tabs, scored 5, non-scored 10,20,40.] ▶LK ♀C (1st trimester) D (2nd & 3rd) ▶? $$

ramipril (*Altace*): HTN: 2.5 mg PO qd, max 20 mg/day. CHF: Start 2.5 mg PO bid, usual dose 5 mg PO bid. [Trade: Caps, 1.25,2.5,5,10.] ▶LK ♀C (1st trimester) D (2nd & 3rd) ◗? $$

trandolapril (*Mavik*): HTN: Start 1 mg PO qd, max 8 mg/day. CHF/post MI: Start 0.5-1 mg PO qd, usual dose 4 mg PO qd. [Trade: Tabs, scored 1, non-scored 2,4.] ▶LK ♀C (1st trimester) D (2nd & 3rd) ◗? $

Angiotensin Receptor Blockers (ARBs) (see also antihypertensive combos)

candesartan (*Atacand*): HTN: Start 16 mg PO qd, maximum 32 mg/day. [Trade: Tabs, non-scored 4,8,16,32.] ▶K ♀C (1st trimester) D (2nd & 3rd) ◗? $$

eprosartan (*Teveten*): HTN: Start 600 mg PO qd, maximum 800 mg/day given qd or divided bid. [Trade: Tablet, scored 400, non-scored 600.] ▶Fecal excretion ♀C (1st trimester) D (2nd & 3rd) ◗? $$

irbesartan (*Avapro*): HTN: Start 150 mg PO qd, maximum 300 mg/day. Start with 75 mg qd if volume depleted. [Trade: Tabs, non-scored 75,150,300.] ▶L ♀C (1st trimester) D (2nd & 3rd) ◗? $$

losartan (*Cozaar*): HTN: Start 50 mg PO qd, maximum 100 mg/day given qd or divided bid. Start with 25 mg qd if volume depletion or history of hepatic impairment. [Trade: Tabs, non-scored 25,50.] ▶L ♀C (1st trimester) D (2nd & 3rd) ◗? $$

telmisartan (*Micardis*): HTN: Start 40 mg PO qd, maximum 80 mg/day. [Trade: Tabs, non-scored 40,80.] ▶L ♀C (1st trimester) D (2nd & 3rd) ◗? $$

valsartan (*Diovan*): HTN: Start 80 mg PO qd, max 320 mg/day. [Trade: Caps 80,160.] ▶L ♀C (1st trimester) D (2nd & 3rd) ◗? $$

Antiadrenergic Agents

clonidine (*Catapres*): HTN: Start 0.1 mg PO bid, max 2.4 mg/day. Can get rebound HTN with abrupt discontinuation, especially at doses ≥ 0.8 mg/d. Transdermal (Catapres-TTS): Start 0.1 mg/24 hour patch q week, titrate to desired effect, max effective dose 0.6 mg/24 hour (two, 0.3 mg/24 hour patches). [Generic/Trade: Tabs, non-scored 0.1,0.2,0.3; Trade only: Patch, 0.1,0.2,0.3 mg/24 hours.] ▶KL ♀C ◗? $

doxazosin (*Cardura*): HTN: Start 1 mg PO qhs, max 16 mg/day. Orthostatic hypotension with initial therapy. [Generic/Trade: Tabs, scored 1,2,4,8.] ▶L ♀C ◗? $$

methyldopa (*Aldomet*): HTN: Start 250 mg PO bid/tid, max 3000 mg/day. May cause hemolytic anemia. [Generic/Trade: Tabs, non-scored 125,250,500.] ▶LK ♀B ◗+ $$

prazosin (*Minipress*): HTN: Start 1 mg PO bid/tid, max 40 mg/day. Take first dose at bedtime to avoid orthostatic hypotension. [Generic/Trade: Caps 1,2,5.] ▶L ♀C ◗? $$

reserpine (*Serpasil*): HTN: Start 0.05-0.1 mg PO qd or 0.1 mg PO qod, max 0.25 mg/day. [Generic: Tabs, scored, 0.1,0.25.] ▶LK ♀C ◗- $

terazosin (*Hytrin*): HTN: Start 1 mg PO qhs, usual effective dose 1-5 mg PO qd or divided bid, max 20 mg/day. Orthostatic hypotension with initial therapy. [Generic (Tabs)/Trade (Caps): 1,2,5,10.] ▶LK ♀C ◗? $$

Anti-Dysrhythmics / Cardiac Arrest

adenosine (*Adenocard*): PSVT conversion (not A-fib): 6 mg rapid IV & flush, preferably through a central line. If no response after 1-2 mins then 12 mg. A third dose of 12-18 mg may be given prn. Peds initial dose 50 mcg/kg, subsequent 100-200 mcg/kg. Half-life is <10 seconds. ▶Plasma ♀C ◗? $$$

amiodarone (*Cordarone, Pacerone*): Life-threatening ventricular arrhythmia: Load 150 mg IV over 10 min, then 1 mg/min x 6h, then 0.5 mg/min x 18h. Mix in D5W. Oral load 800-1600 mg PO qd for 1-3 wks, reduce to 400-800 mg PO qd for 1 month when arrhythmia is controlled, reduce to lowest effective dose thereafter, usually 200-400 mg qd. Photosensitivity with oral therapy. Pulmonary toxicity. May increase digoxin levels by 70%. Significantly increases INR with warfarin. IV therapy may cause hypotension. Contraindicated with marked bradycardia or heart block without pacemaker. [Generic/Trade: Tabs, scored 200.] ▶L ♀D ◗- $$$$

atropine: Bradyarrhythmia/CPR: 0.5-1.0 mg IV/ET. Peds: 0.02 mg/kg/dose, minimum 0.1 mg total dose. ▶K ♀C ◗- $

bicarbonate sodium: Severe acidosis: 1 mEq/kg up to 50-100 mEq/dose IV. ▶K ♀C ◗? $

bretylium (*Bretylol, Bretylate*): Ventricular arrhythmia: Initial 5 mg/kg IV, then 10 mg/kg if needed. Infusion 500 mg in 50mL D5W (10 mg/mL) at 1-3 mg/min (7-21 mL/h). ▶K ♀C ◗? $$

digoxin (*Lanoxin, Lanoxicaps, Digitek*): Atrial fibrillation/CHF: 0.125-0.25 mg PO qd. Rapid A-fib: Load 0.5 mg IV, then 0.25 mg IV q6h x 2 doses, maintenance 0.125-0.375 mg IV/PO qd. [Generic/Trade: Tabs, scored (Lanoxin) 0.125,0.25, 0.5; Trade only: Caps (Lanoxicaps), 0.05,0.1,0.2; Generic/Trade: elixir 0.05 mg/mL.] ▶KL ♀C ◗+ $

digoxin-immune Fab (*Digibind*): Dig toxicity: 2-20 vials IV, one formula is: Number vials = (serum dig level in ng/mL) x (kg) / 100. ▶K ♀C ◗? $$$$$

dofetilide (*Tikosyn*): A-fib/flutter: Specialized dosing based on creatinine clearance and QTc interval. [Trade: Caps, 0.125,0.25,0.5.] ▶KL ♀C ◗- $$$$

epinephrine: Cardiac arrest: 0.5 - 1 mg IV/ET; Anaphylaxis: 0.1-0.5 mg SC/IM, may repeat SC dose every 10-15 minutes. EpiPen Auto-injector delivers 0.3 mg (1:1,000 soln) IM dose. ▶Plasma ♀C ◗- $

ibutilide (*Corvert*): A-fib/flutter: 0.01 mg/kg up to 1 mg IV over 10 mins, may repeat if no response after 10 more minutes. Torsade de pointes in up to 8%, keep on cardiac monitor at least 4 hours. ▶K ♀C ◗? $$$$$

isoproterenol (*Isuprel*): Refractory bradycardia or third degree AV block: 2 mg in 250mL D5W (8 mcg/mL) at 5 mcg/min. 5 mcg/min = 37 mL/h. Peds: 0.1-1.0 mcg/kg/min. 10 kg: 0.1 mcg/kg/min = 8 mL/h. ▶LK ♀C ◗? $$

lidocaine (*Xylocaine, Xylocard*): Ventricular arrhythmia: Load 1 mg/kg IV, then 0.5 mg/kg q8-10min as needed to max 3 mg/kg. IV infusion: 4 gm in 500 ml D5W (8 mg/ml) at 1-4 mg/min. Peds: 20-50 mcg/kg/min. ▶LK ♀B ◗? $

procainamide (*Procanbid, Pronestyl*): Ventricular arrhythmia: 500-1250 mg PO q6h or 50 mg/kg/day. Extended-release: 500-1000 mg PO q12h. Load 100 mg IV q10min or 20 mg/min (150 mL/h) until: 1) QRS widens >50%, 2) dysrhythmia suppressed, 3) hypotension, or 4) total of 17 mg/kg or 1000 mg. Infusion 2g in 250mL D5W (8 mg/mL) at 2-6 mg/min (15-45 mL/h). [Generic/Trade: Tabs, immediate-release, non-scored and Caps (Pronestyl) 250,375,500; Generic only: Tabs, sustained release, non-scored (generic procainamide SR, q6h dosing), 250,500,750; Trade only: Tabs, extended-release, non-scored (Procanbid, q12h dosing) 500,1000.] ▶LK ♀C ◗- $$$

quinidine gluconate (*Quinaglute, Quinalan, Quinate*): A-fib/flutter, ventricular premature complexes: 324-648 mg PO q8-12h. [Generic/Trade: Tabs, extended-release, non-scored (Quinaglute) 324, scored (Quinalan) 324.] ▶LK ♀C ◗- $$

quinidine sulfate (*Quinidex, Quinora*): A-fib/flutter: Immediate-release: 200-400 mg PO 6-8h. Extended-release: 300-600 mg PO q8-12h. [Generic/Trade: Tabs, non-scored immediate-release 200,300 (Quinora); Generic/Trade: Tabs, extended-release 300 (Quinidex Extentabs).] ▶LK ♀C ◗- $

sotalol (*Betapace, Betapace AF, Rylosol, Sotacar*): Ventricular arrhythmia: Start 80 mg PO bid, max 640 mg/d. Caution – higher incidence of torsades with >320 mg/day, women, and CHF. [Generic/Trade: Tabs, scored 80,120,160,240; Trade only: 80,120, 160 (Betapace AF)] ▶K ♀B ▶- $$$$

Anti-Hyperlipidemic Agents - Bile Acid Sequestrants

cholestyramine (*Questran, Questran Light, Prevalite, LoCHOLEST, LoCHOLEST Light*): Elevated LDL cholesterol: Powder: Start 4 g PO qd/bid before meals, increase up to max 36 g/day. [Generic/Trade: Powder for oral susp, 4 g cholestyramine resin / 9 g powder (Questran, LoCHOLEST), 4 g cholestyramine resin / 5 g powder (Questran Light, LoCHOLEST Light) 4 g cholestyramine resin / 5.5 g powder (Prevalite).] ▶Fecal excretion ♀C ▶+ $$

colesevelam (*Welchol*): Elevated LDL cholesterol: 3 Tabs bid with meals or 6 Tabs once daily with a meal, max dose 7 Tabs/day. [Trade: Tabs, non-scored, 625.] ▶Not absorbed ♀B ▶+

colestipol (*Colestid, Colestid Flavored*): Elevated LDL cholesterol: Tabs: Start 2 g PO qd/bid, max 16 g/day. Granules: Start 5 g PO qd/bid, max 30 g/day. [Trade: Tabs, 1 g; Trade: Granules for oral susp, 5 g / 7.5 g powder.] ▶Fecal excretion ♀B ▶+ $$$

Anti-Hyperlipidemic Agents - HMG-CoA Reductase Inhibitors ("Statins")

atorvastatin (*Lipitor*): Hypercholesterolemia: Start 10 mg PO qd, max 80 mg/day. [Trade: Tabs, non-scored 10,20,40,80.] ▶L ♀X ▶- $$$

cerivastatin (*Baycol*): Hypercholesterolemia: 0.4 mg PO qpm, 0.2 mg if renal impairment. Max 0.8 mg/day. [Trade: Tabs, non-scored 0.2,0.3,0.4,0.8.] ▶LK ♀X ▶- $$

fluvastatin (*Lescol*): Hypercholesterolemia: Start 20-40 mg PO qhs, max 80 mg/day. Divide bid if 80 mg/day. [Trade: Caps, 20,40.] ▶L ♀X ▶- $$

lovastatin (*Mevacor*): Hypercholesterolemia: Start 20 mg PO qpm, max 80 mg/day qd or divided bid. [Trade: Tabs, non-scored 10,20,40.] ▶L ♀X ▶- $$$

pravastatin (*Pravachol*): Hypercholesterolemia: Start 10-20 mg PO qd, max 40 mg/d. [Trade: Tabs, non-scored 10,20,40.] ▶L ♀X ▶- $$$

simvastatin (*Zocor*): Hypercholesterolemia: Start 20-40 mg PO qpm, max 80 mg/d. [Trade: Tabs, non-scored 5,10,20,40,80.] ▶L ♀X ▶- $$$$

LIPID RESPONSE* *(%change)*	*Cholesterol*	*LDL**	*HDL**	*Triglycerides*	***LFT MONITORING FOR STATINS****
atorvastatin 10 mg	-29%	-39%	+6%	-19%	B, 12 wk, semiannually
cerivastatin 0.4 mg	-24%	-34%	+7%	-16%	B, 6 & 12 wk, semiannually
fluvastatin 40 mg	-19%	-25%	+4%	-14%	B, 12 wk
lovastatin 20 mg	-17%	-24%	+7%	-10%	B, 6 & 12 wk, semiannually
pravastatin 20 mg	-24%	-32%	+2%	-11%	B, 12 wk
simvastatin 20 mg	-28%	-38%	+8%	-15%	B, 6 mo, 12 mo ***

*Data taken from prescribing info at recommended starting doses. **Schedule for LFT monitoring when starting therapy and after each dosage increase. Stop statin therapy if LFTs are > 3x upper limit of normal. B = baseline, LDL = low-density lipoprotein, HDL = high-density lipoprotein, ***For first year only or after last dose increase. Get LFTs 3,6,12 months after increase to 80 mg.

Anti-Hyperlipidemic Agents - Other

fenofibrate (*Tricor*): Hypertriglyceridemia: Start 67 mg (1 capsule) PO qd with a meal. Max 200 mg qd. [Trade: Capsule, 67,134,200.] ▶LK ♀C ▶- $$$

gemfibrozil (*Lopid*): Hypertriglyceridemia: 600 mg PO bid. [Generic/Trade: Tabs, scored 600.] ▶LK ♀C ▶? $$

niacin (*nicotinic acid, vitamin B3, Niacor, Nicolar, Niaspan*): Hyperlipidemia: Start 50-100 mg PO bid/tid with meals & increase slowly as tolerated until approx 1.5-3 g/day, max 6 g/d. Extended-release (Niaspan): Titration starter pack for wks 1-3, then 1000 mg PO qhs for wks 4-7, then titrate to response. Extended-release formulations not listed here may have greater hepatotoxicity. [Generic (OTC): Tabs, scored 25,50,100,150,500; ext-release, non-scored (Niaspan), 500,750,1000.] ▶K ♀C ▶? $

omega-3 fatty acid (fish oil) (*Promega, Cardio-Omega 3, Sea-Omega, Marine Lipid Concentrate, SuperEPA 1200*): Hypertriglyceridemia: 3-5 gm EPA+DHA content daily. Marine Lipid Concentrate, Super EPA 1200 mg capsule contains EPA 360 mg + DHA 240 mg, daily dose = 5-8 Caps. [Trade/Generic: Capsule, shown as EPA+DHA mg content, 240 (Promega Pearls), 300 (Cardi-Omega 3, Max EPA), 400 (Promega), 500 (Sea-Omega), 600 (Marine Lipid Concentrate, SuperEPA 1200), 875 (SuperEPA 2000).] ▶L ♀? ▶? $$

Antihypertensive Combinations

NOTE: Dosage should first be adjusted by using each drug separately.

Accuretic (quinapril/HCTZ): [Trade: Tabs 10/12.5, 20/12.5, 20/25.]; *Aldactazide* (spironolactone/HCTZ): [Generic/Trade: Tabs 25/25, scored 50/50.]; *Apresazide* (hydralazine/HCTZ): [Generic/Trade: Caps 25/25, 50/50, Trade only: Caps 100/50.]; *Avalide* (irbesartan/HCTZ): [Trade: Tabs 150/12.5, 300/12.5.]; *Capozide* (captopril/HCTZ): [Generic/Trade: Tabs scored 25/15, 25/ 25, 50/15, 50/25.]; *Combipres* (clonidine/chlorthalidone): [Generic/Trade: Tabs 0.1/15, 0.2/15, 0.3/15.]; *Corzide* (nadolol/bendroflumethlazide): [Trade: Tabs scored 40/5, 80/5.]; *Diovan HCT* (valsartan/HCTZ): [Trade: Tabs 80/12.5, 160/12.5.]; *Dyazide* (triamterene/HCTZ): [Generic/Trade: Caps (Dyazide) 37.5/25, (generic only) 50/25.]; *Hyzaar* (losartan/HCTZ): [Trade: Tabs 50/12.5, 100/25.]; *Inderide* (propranolol/HCTZ): [Generic/Trade: Tabs scored 40/25, 80/25.]; *Inderide LA* (propranolol/HCTZ): [Generic/Trade:Caps extended-release 80/50, 120/ 50, 160/50]; *Lexxel* (enalapril/felodipine): [Trade: Tabs 5/2.5, 5/5.]; *Lopressor HCT* (metoprolol/HCTZ): [Trade: Tabs scored 50/25, 100/25, 100/50.]; *Lotensin HCT* (benazepril/HCTZ): [Trade: Tabs 5/6.25, 10/12.5, 20/12.5, 20/25.]; *Lotrel* (amlodipine/benazepril): [Trade: Capsule, 2.5/10, 5/10, 5 /20]; *Maxzide* (triamterene/HCTZ): [Generic/Trade: Tabs scored (Maxzide-25) 37.5/25 (Maxzide) 75/50]; *Maxzide-25* (triamterene/HCTZ): [Generic/Trade: Tabs scored (Maxzide-25) 37.5/25 (Maxzide) 75/50.]; *Minizide* (prazosin/polythiazide): [Trade: Capsule 1/0.5, 2/0.5, 5/0.5]; *Moduretic, Moduret* (amiloride/HCTZ). [Generic/Trade: Tabs scored 5/50.]; *Prinzide* (lisinopril/HCTZ): [Trade: Tabs 10/12.5, 20/12.5, 20/25.]; *Tarka* (trandolapril/verapamil): [Trade: Tabs 2/180, 1/240, 2/240, 4/240.]; *Tenoretic* (atenolol/chlorthalidone): [Generic/Trade: Tabs scored 50/25, 100/25.]; *Timolide* (timolol/HCTZ): [Trade: Tabs 10/25.]; *Uniretic* (moexipril/HCTZ): [Trade: Tabs scored 7.5/12.5, 15/25.]; *Vaseretic* (enalapril/HCTZ): [Generic/Trade: Tabs 5/12.5, 10/25.]; *Zestoretic* (lisinopril/HCTZ): [Trade: Tabs 10/12.5, 20/12.5, 20/25.]; *Ziac* (bisoprolol/HCTZ): [Trade: Tabs 2.5/6.25, 5/6.25, 10/6.25.]

Antihypertensives - Miscellaneous

hydralazine (*Apresoline*): Hypertensive emergency: 10-50 mg IM or 10-20 mg IV, repeat prn. HTN: Start 10 mg PO tid/qid, max 400 mg/day. Headaches, peripheral edema, lupus syndrome. [Generic/Trade: Tabs 10,25,50,100.] ▶LK ♀C ▶+ $

minoxidil (*Loniten*): Refractory HTN: Start 2.5-5 mg PO qd, max 100 mg/day. [Generic/Trade: Tabs, scored, 2.5,10.] ▶K ♀C ▶- $$

nitroprusside sodium (*Nipride, Nitropress*): Hypertensive emergency: 50 mg in 250 mL D5W (200 mcg/mL), start at 0.3 mcg/kg/min (for 70 kg adult = 6 mL/h). Max 10 mcg/kg/min. Cyanide toxicity with high doses and prolonged infusions, check thiocyanate levels. ▶RBC's ♀C ▶- $

phentolamine (*Regitine, Rogitine*): Diagnosis of pheochromocytoma: 5 mg increments IV. Peds 0.1 mg/kg up to 5 mg per dose. Extravasation: 5-10 mg in 10 mL NS local injection. ▶Plasma ♀C ▶? $$

Antiplatelet Drugs

abciximab (*ReoPro*): Platelet aggregation inhibition, percutaneous coronary intervention: 0.25 mg/kg IV bolus via separate infusion line before procedure, then 0.125 mcg/kg/min (max 10 mcg/min) IV infusion x 12h. ▶Plasma ♀C ▶? $$$$$

Aggrenox (dipyridamole/aspirin): Platelet aggregation inhibition: 1 capsule bid. [Trade: Caps, 200/25.] ▶LK ♀D ▶? $$$

anagrelide (*Agrylin*): Essential thrombocythemia: Start 0.5 mg PO qid or 1 mg PO bid, then after 1 week adjust to lowest effective dose. Max 10 mg/d. [Trade: Caps, 0.5,1.] ▶LK ♀C ▶? $$$$$

aspirin (*Ecotrin, Empirin, Halfprin, Bayer, ASA, Entrophen*): Platelet aggregation inhibition: 81-325 mg PO qd. [Generic/Trade (OTC): Tabs, 325,500; chewable 81; enteric 81,165 (Halfprin), 81,325,500 (Ecotrin), 650,975; Trade only: controlled-release 650,800 (ZORprin, Rx); Generic only (OTC): Supp 120,200,300,600.] ▶K ♀D ▶? $

clopidogrel (*Plavix*): Platelet aggregation inhibition: 75 mg PO qd. Rare TTP. [Trade: Tabs, non-scored 75.] ▶LK ♀B ▶? $$$

dipyridamole (*Persantine*): Antithrombotic: 75-100 mg PO qid. [Generic/Trade: Tabs, non-scored 25,50,75.] ▶L ♀B ▶? $$

eptifibatide (*Integrilin*): Acute coronary syndromes: Load 180 mcg/kg, then infusion 2 mcg/kg/min x 72 hours. Percutaneous cardiovascular intervention: Load 135 mcg/kg IV bolus just before procedure, then IV infusion 0.5 mcg/kg/min x 20-24 hours after procedure. ▶K ♀B ▶? $$$$$

ticlopidine (*Ticlid*): Due to adverse effects, other drugs preferred. Platelet aggregation inhibition/reduction of thrombotic stroke: 250 mg PO bid with food. Neutropenia, TTP. [Generic/Trade: Tabs, non-scored 250.] ▶L ♀B ▶? $$$$

tirofiban (*Aggrastat*): Acute coronary syndromes: Start 0.4 mcg/kg/min x 30 mins, then decrease to 0.1 mcg/kg/min x 48-108 hours or until 12-24 hours after coronary intervention. Half dose with CrCl < 30 mL/min. Use concurrent heparin to keep PTT twice normal. ▶K ♀B ▶? $$$$$

Beta Blockers (see also antihypertensive combos)

acebutolol (*Sectral, Monitan*): HTN: Start 400 mg PO qd or 200 mg PO bid, max 1200 mg/day. Beta1 receptor selective. [Generic/Trade: Caps, 200,400.] ▶LK ♀B ▶- $$

atenolol (*Tenormin*): Acute MI: 5 mg IV over 5 min, repeat in 10 min. HTN: Start 25-50 mg PO qd or divided bid, maximum 100 mg/day. Beta1 receptor selective. [Generic/Trade: Tabs, non-scored 25,100; scored, 50.] ▶K ♀D ▶- $

betaxolol (*Kerlone*): HTN: Start 5-10 mg PO qd, max 20 mg/day. Beta1 receptor selective. [Generic/Trade: Tabs, scored 10, non-scored 20.] ▶LK ♀C ▶? $

bisoprolol (*Zebeta*): HTN: Start 2.5-5 mg PO qd, max 20 mg/day. Beta1 receptor selective. [Trade: Tabs, scored 5, non-scored 10.] ▶LK ♀C ◗? $$

carvedilol (*Coreg*): CHF: Start 3.125 mg PO bid with food, double dose q2 weeks as tolerated up to max of 25 mg bid (if <85 kg) or 50 mg bid (if >85 kg). HTN: Start 6.25 mg PO bid, max 50 mg/day. Beta1 and beta2 receptor blocker. Not first line agent for HTN. Alpha1, beta1, and beta2 receptor blocker. [Trade: Tabs, non-scored 3.125, scored, 6.25, 12.5,25.] ▶L ♀C ◗? $$$

esmolol (*Brevibloc*): SVT/HTN emergency: Mix infusion 5g in 500mL (10 mg/mL), load with 500 mcg/kg over 1 minute (70 kg: 35 mg or 3.5 mL) then infusion 50-200 mcg/kg/min. 70 kg: 100 mcg/kg/min = 40 mL/h. Half-life=9 min. Beta1 selective. ▶K ♀C ◗?

labetalol (*Trandate, Normodyne*): HTN: Start 100 mg PO bid, max 2400 mg/day. HTN emergency: Start 20 mg IV slow injection, then 40-80 mg IV q10 min prn up to 300 mg or IV infusion 0.5-2 mg/min. Peds: Start 0.3-1 mg/kg/dose (max 20 mg). Alpha1, beta1, and beta2 receptor blocker. [Generic/Trade: Tabs, scored 100,200 (Trandate, Normodyne), 300 (Trandate); non-scored 300 (Normodyne).] ▶LK ♀C ◗+ $$

metoprolol (*Lopressor, Toprol XL, Betaloc*): Acute MI: 5 mg increments IV q5-15 min up to 15 mg followed by oral therapy if tolerated. HTN: Start 25-50 mg PO bid or 50-100 mg PO qd (extended-release), max 450 mg/day. Beta1 receptor selective. [Generic/Trade: Tabs, scored 50,100; Trade only: extended-release Tabs, scored (Toprol XL) 50,100,200.] ▶L ♀C ◗? $$

nadolol (*Corgard*): HTN: Start 20-40 mg PO qd, max 320 mg/day. Beta1 and beta2 receptor blocker. [Generic/Trade: Tabs, scored 20,40,80,120,160.] ▶K ♀C ◗- $$

pindolol (*Visken*): HTN: Start 5 mg PO bid, max 60 mg/day. Beta1 and beta2 receptor blocker. [Generic/Trade: Tabs, scored 5,10.] ▶K ♀B ◗? $$$

propranolol (*Inderal*): HTN: Start 20-40 mg PO bid, max 640 mg/d; extended-release: Start 60-80 mg PO qd, max 640 mg/day. Life-threatening arrhythmia: 1 mg IV increments q2min. Beta 1&2 blocker. [Generic/Trade: Tabs, scored 10,20,40,60,80, Generic only: Tabs, 90; Generic/Trade: solution, 20,40 mg/5mL, concentrate, 80 mg/mL; Generic/Trade: Caps, extended-release, 60,80,120,160.] ▶L ♀C ◗+ $

timolol (*Blocadren*): HTN: Start 10 mg PO bid, max 60 mg/d. Beta1 and beta2 receptor blocker. [Generic/Trade: Tabs, non-scored 5, scored 10,20.] ▶LK ♀C ◗? $$

Calcium Channel Blockers (CCBs) - Dihydropyridines

amlodipine (*Norvasc*): HTN: Start 2.5 to 5 mg PO qd, max 10 qd. [Trade: Tabs, non-scored 2.5,5,10.] ▶L ♀C ◗? $$

felodipine (*Plendil, Renedil*): HTN: Start 5 mg PO qd, maximum 20 mg/d. [Trade: Tabs, extended-release, non-scored 2.5,5,10.] ▶L ♀C ◗? $$

isradipine (*DynaCirc, DynaCirc CR*): HTN: Start 2.5 mg PO bid, max 20 mg/day (max 10 mg/day in elderly). Controlled-release: 5-10 mg PO qd. [Trade: Caps, 2.5,5, controlled-release Tabs, non-scored 5,10.] ▶L ♀C ◗? $$$

nicardipine (*Cardene*): HTN emergency: Begin IV infusion at 5 mg/h, titrate to effect, max 15 mg/h. HTN: Start 20 mg PO tid, max 120 mg/day. Sustained release: Start 30 mg PO bid, max 120 mg/day. [Generic/Trade: Caps, immediate-release 20,30, Trade only: sustained-release 30,45,60.] ▶L ♀C ◗? $$

nifedipine (*Procardia XL, Adalat CC*): HTN/angina: extended-release: 30-60 mg PO qd, max 120/d. Angina: immediate-release: Start 10 mg PO tid, max 120 mg/d. Avoid SL administration, may cause excessive hypotension, stroke. Do not use immediate-release caps for treating HTN. [Generic/Trade: Caps, 10,20; Generic/Trade: Tabs, extended-release, non-scored 30,60,90.] ▶L ♀C ◗+ $$

nisoldipine (*Sular*): HTN: Start 20 mg PO qd, max 60 mg/day. Avoid concomitant grapefruit and grapefruit juice, which may significantly enhance effect. [Trade: Tabs, extended-release, non-scored 10,20,30,40.] ▶L ♀C ▶? $$

Calcium Channel Blockers (CCBs) – Other (see antihypertensive combos)

diltiazem (*Cardizem, Diltia XT, Tiazac, Dilacor, Tiamate*): Rapid atrial fibrillation: bolus 20 mg (0.25 mg/kg) IV over 2 min. Rebolus 15 min later (if needed) 25 mg (0.35 mg/kg). Infusion 5-15 mg/h. HTN: Once daily, extended-release: Start 120-240 mg PO qd, max 540 mg/day. Twice daily, sustained-release: Start 60-120 mg PO bid, max 360 mg/day. Angina: immediate-release, Start 30 mg PO qid, max 360 mg/day divided tid/qid; extended-release, Start 120-240 mg PO qd, max 540 mg/day. [Generic/Trade: Tabs, immediate-release, non-scored (Cardizem) 30, scored 60,90, 120, Trade only: Tabs, extended-release (Tiamate qd) 120; Generic/Trade: Caps, sustained-release (Cardizem SR q12h) 60,90,120, extended-release (Cardizem CD qd) 120,180,240,300,360 Trade only: (Tiazac qd) 120,180,240,300,360,420, (Dilacor XR, Diltia XT qd) 120,180,240.] ▶L ♀C ▶+ $$

verapamil (*Isoptin, Calan, Covera-HS, Verelan PM, Chronovera*): SVT: 5-10 mg IV over 2 min. Peds (>2 yo): 0.075-0.15 mg/kg IV over 2 min. Angina: immediate-release, start 40-80 mg PO tid/qid, max 480 mg/day divided tid/qid; sustained-release, start 120-240 mg PO qd, max 480 mg/day (use bid dosing for doses > 240 mg/day with Isoptin SR and Calan SR); (Covera-HS) 180 mg PO qhs, max 480 mg/day. HTN: same as angina, except (Verelan PM) 100-200 mg PO qhs, max 400 mg/day and immediate-release Tabs should be avoided in treating HTN. [Generic/Trade: Tabs, immediate-release, scored 40,80,120; sustained-release, non-scored (Calan SR, Isoptin SR) 120, scored 180,240; Caps, sustained-release (Verelan) 120,180,240, 360. Trade only: Tabs, extended-release (Covera HS) 180,240; Caps, extended-release (Verelan PM) 100,200,300.] ▶L ♀C ▶+ $$

Diuretics - Carbonic Anhydrase Inhibitors

acetazolamide (*Diamox*): Altitude sickness: 0.5-1 gm PO divided bid-tid or sustained-release 500 mg PO qd-bid beginning 24-48hr before ascent and for 48hr at high altitude. [Generic/Trade: Tabs, 125,250; Trade only: capsule, sustained-release, 500.] ▶LK ♀C ▶+ $$

Diuretics - Loop

bumetanide (*Bumex*): Edema: 0.5-1 mg IV/IM. 0.5-2 mg PO qd. 1 mg bumetanide is roughly equivalent to 40 mg furosemide. [Generic/Trade: Tabs, scored 0.5,1,2.] ▶K ♀C ▶? $

ethacrynic acid (*Edecrin*): Rarely used. 0.5-1.0 mg/kg up to 50 mg IV. 25-100 mg PO qd/bid. [Trade: Tabs, scored 25,50.] ▶K ♀B ▶? $$

furosemide (*Lasix*): Edema: Initial dose 20-80 mg IV/IM/PO, increase dose by 20-40 mg every 6-8h until desired response is achieved, max 600 mg/day. [Generic/Trade: Tabs, non-scored 20, scored 40,80; Generic/Trade: oral solution 10 mg/mL, 40 mg/5mL.] ▶K ♀C ▶? $

torsemide (*Demadex*): Edema: 5-20 mg IV/PO qd. [Trade: Tabs, scored 5,10,20,100.] ▶LK ♀B ▶? $

Diuretics - Potassium Sparing (see also antihypertensive combos)

amiloride (*Midamor*): Diuretic-induced hypokalemia: 5 mg PO qd, max 20 mg/day. [Generic/Trade: Tabs, non-scored 5.] ▶LK ♀B ▶? $$

spironolactone (*Aldactone*): HTN/edema: 50-100 mg PO qd or divided bid. CHF: 25-50 mg PO qd. [Generic/Trade: Tabs, non-scored 25; scored 50,100.] ▶LK ♀D ▶+ $

Diuretics - Thiazide Type (see also antihypertensive combos)

chlorothiazide (*Diuril*): HTN: 125-250 mg PO qd or divided bid, max 1000 mg/day. Edema: 500-2000 mg PO/IV qd or divided bid. [Generic/Trade: Tabs, scored 250,500; Trade only: susp, 250 mg/5mL.] ▶L ♀B ▶+ $

chlorthalidone (*Hygroton, Thalitone*): HTN: 12.5-25 mg PO qd, max 50 mg/day. Edema: 50-100 mg PO qd, max 200 mg/day. [Trade only: Tabs, non-scored (Thalitone) 15; Generic/Trade: Tabs, non-scored (Thalitone, Hygroton) 25,50, scored (Hygroton) 100.] ▶L ♀B ▶+ $

hydrochlorothiazide (*HCTZ, Oretic, HydroDIURIL, Esidrix, Microzide*): HTN: 12.5-25 mg PO qd, max 50 mg/day. Edema: 25-100 mg PO qd, max 200 mg/day. [Generic/Trade: Tabs, scored 25,50,100; cap, 12.5; solution, 50 mg/5mL, concentrate, 100 mg/mL.] ▶L ♀B ▶+ $

indapamide (*Lozol*): HTN: 1.25-5 mg PO qd, max 5 mg/day. Edema: 2.5-5 mg PO qam. [Generic/Trade: Tabs, non-scored 1.25, 2.5.] ▶L ♀B ▶? $

metolazone (*Zaroxolyn, Mykrox*): Zaroxolyn: 2.5-5 mg PO qd for HTN; 5-20 mg qd for CHF. Mykrox: 0.5-1 mg qd for HTN. [Trade: Tabs, non-scored (Mykrox) 0.5, (Zaroxolyn) 2.5,5,10.] ▶L ♀B ▶? $

Nitrates

isosorbide dinitrate (*Isordil, Sorbitrate, Dilatrate-SR*): Angina prophylaxis: 5-40 mg PO 3 tid (7 am, noon, & 5 pm), sustained-release: 40-80 mg PO bid (8 am & 2 pm). Acute angina attack, sublingual Tabs: 2.5-10 mg SL q5-10 min prn, up to 3 doses in 30 min. [Generic/Trade: Tabs, scored 5,10,20,30,40, chewable, scored 5,10, sustained-release, scored 40, sublingual Tabs, non-scored 2.5,5,10; Trade only: capsule, sustained-release (Dilatrate-SR, Isordil Tembids) 40.] ▶L ♀C ▶? $

isosorbide mononitrate (*ISMO, Monoket, Imdur*): Angina: 20 mg PO twice daily (8 am and 3 pm). Extended-release: Start 30-60 mg PO qd, maximum 240 mg/day. [Generic/Trade: Tabs, non-scored (ISMO) 20, scored (Monoket) 10,20, extended-release, scored (Imdur) 30,60, non-scored 120.] ▶L ♀C ▶? $$

nitroglycerin intravenous infusion (*Tridil, NitroBid IV*): Perioperative HTN, acute MI/CHF, acute angina: mix 50 mg in 250 mL D5W (200 mcg/mL), start at 10-20 mcg/min (3-6 mL/h), then titrate upward by 5-20 mcg/min as needed. ▶L ♀C ▶? $

nitroglycerin ointment (*Nitrol, Nitro-bid*): Angina prophylaxis: Start 0.5 inch q8h, maintenance 1-2 inches q8h, max 4 inches q4-6h; 15 mg/inch. Allow for a nitrate-free period of 10-14h to avoid nitrate tolerance. [Generic/Trade: Ointment, 2%.] ▶L ♀C ▶? $

nitroglycerin spray (*Nitrolingual*): Acute angina: 1-2 sprays under the tongue prn, max 3 sprays in 15 min. [Trade: Solution, 0.4 mg/spray (200 sprays/canister).] ▶L ♀C ▶? $$

nitroglycerin sublingual (*Nitrostat, NitroQuick*): Acute angina: 0.4 mg SL under tongue, repeat dose every 5 min as needed up to 3 doses in 15 min. [Trade: Sublingual Tabs, non-scored 0.3,0.4,0.6; in bottles of 100 or package of 4 bottles with 25 Tabs each.] ▶L ♀C ▶? $

nitroglycerin sustained release (*Nitrong, Nitroglyn*): Angina prophylaxis: Start 2.5 or 2.6 mg PO bid/tid, then titrate upward prn. Allow for a nitrate-free period of 10-14h to avoid tolerance. [Trade only: Tabs, scored, extended-release (Nitrong) 2.6,6.5,9; Generic/Trade: capsule, extended-release (Nitroglyn) 2.5,6.5,9,13.5.] ▶L ♀C ◗? $

nitroglycerin transdermal (*Deponit, Minitran, Nitrodisc, Nitro-Dur, Transderm-Nitro, Trinipatch*): Angina prophylaxis: 1 patch 12-14 hours each day. Allow for a nitrate-free period of 10-14 hours each day to avoid nitrate tolerance. [Trade: Transdermal system, doses in mg/h: Nitro-Dur 0.1,0.2,0.3,0.4,0.6,0.8; Minitran 0.1,0.2,0.4,0.6; Nitrodisc 0.2,0.3,0.4; Deponit 0.2,0.4; Transderm-Nitro 0.1,0.2,0.4,0.6,0.8; Generic only: Transdermal system, doses in mg/h: 0.2,0.4,0.6.] ▶L ♀C ◗? $$

Pressors / Inotropes

dobutamine (*Dobutrex*): Inotropic support: 250 mg in 250mL D5W (1 mg/mL) at 2-20 mcg/kg/min. 70 kg: 5 mcg/kg/min = 21 mL/h. ▶Plasma ♀D ◗- $

dopamine (*Intropin*): Pressor: 400 mg in 250mL D5W (1600 mcg/mL) start at 5 mcg/kg/min, increase as needed by 5-10 mcg/kg/min increments at 10 min intervals, max 50 mcg/kg/min. 70 kg: 5 mcg/kg/min = 13 mL/h. Doses in mcg/kg/min: 2-5 = (renal dose, if no change in pulse or BP) dopaminergic receptors; 5-10 = (cardiac dose) dopaminergic & beta1; >10 = dopaminergic, beta1, & alpha1. ▶Plasma ♀C ◗- $

ephedrine: Pressor: 10-25 mg slow IV, repeat q5-10 min prn. ▶K ♀C ◗? $

epinephrine: Cardiac arrest: 1 mg IV/ET. Anaphylaxis: 0.1-0.5 mg SC/IM, may repeat SC dose q 10-15 minutes. IV Infusion: 1 mg in 250 mL D5W (4 mcg/mL) at 1-4 mcg/min (15-60 mL/h). ▶Plasma ♀C ◗- $

midodrine (*ProAmatine*): Orthostatic hypotension: 10 mg PO tid while awake. [Trade: Tabs, scored 2.5,5.] ▶LK ♀C ◗? $$$$$

milrinone (*Primacor*): CHF (NYHA class III,IV): Load 50 mcg/kg IV over 10 min, then begin IV infusion of 0.375-0.75 mcg/kg/min. ▶K ♀C ◗? $$$$$

norepinephrine (*Levophed*): Acute hypotension: 4 mg in 500 mL D5W (8 mcg/mL) start 8-12 mcg/min, adjust to maintain BP, average maintenance rate 2-4 mcg/min, ideally through central line. 3 mcg/min = 20 mL/h. ▶Plasma ♀C ◗? $

phenylephrine (*Neo-Synephrine*): Severe hypotension: 50 mcg boluses IV. Infusion: 20 mg in 250mL D5W (80 mcg/mL), start 100-180 mcg/min (75-135 mL/h), usual dose once BP is stabilized 40-60 mcg/min. ▶Plasma ♀C ◗- $$$

Thrombolytics

alteplase (*t-PA, Activase*): Acute MI: 15 mg IV bolus, then 50 mg over 30 min, then 35 mg over the next 60 min; (patient ≤67 kg) 15 mg IV bolus, then 0.75 mg/kg (max 50 mg) over 30 min, then 0.5 mg/kg (max 35 mg) over the next 60 min. Concurrent heparin infusion. Acute pulmonary embolism: 100 mg IV over 2h, then restart heparin when PTT ≤twice normal. ▶L ♀C ◗? $$$$$

reteplase (*Retavase*): Acute MI: 10.8 units IV over 2 min; repeat in 30 min. ▶L ♀C ◗? $$$$$

streptokinase (*Streptase, Kabikinase*): Acute MI: 1.5 million units IV over 60 minutes. ▶L ♀C ◗? $$$$$

tenecteplase (*TNKase*): Acute MI: Single IV bolus dose over 5 seconds based on body weight; < 60 kg, 30 mg; 60-69 kg, 35 mg; 70-79 kg, 40 mg; 80-89 kg, 45 mg; ≥90kg, 50 mg. ▶L ♀C ◗? $$$$$

Volume Expanders

albumin (*Albuminar, Buminate, Albumarc*): Shock, burns: 500 mL of 5% solution IV infusion as rapidly as tolerated, repeat in 30 min if needed. ▶L ♀C ▶? $$$$

dextran (*Rheomacrodex, Gentran, Macrodex*): Shock/hypovolemia: 20 mL/kg up to 500 mL IV. ▶K ♀C ▶? $$$$

hetastarch (*Hespan, Hextend*): Shock/hypovolemia: 500-1000 mL IV 6% solution. ▶K ♀C ▶? $$

plasma protein fraction (*Plasmanate, Protenate, Plasmatein*): Shock/hypovolemia. 5% sol'n 250-500 mL IV prn. ▶L ♀C ▶? $$$$

CONTRAST MEDIA

NOTE: Beware of allergic or anaphylactoid reactions. Avoid in renal insufficiency or dehydration. Hold metformin (*Glucophage*) prior to or at the time of iodinated contrast dye use and for 48h after procedure. Restart after procedure only if renal function is normal.

barium sulfate: Non-iodinated GI (eg, oral, rectal) contrast. ▶Not absorbed ♀? ▶+ $

diatrizoate (*Hypaque, Renografin, Gastrografin, MD-Gastroview, Cystografin*): Iodinated, ionic, high osmolality IV or GI contrast. ▶K ♀C ▶? $

gadodiamide (*Omniscan*): Non-iodinated, non-ionic IV contrast for MRI. ▶K ♀C ▶? $$$$

gadopentetate (*Magnevist*): Non-iodinated IV contrast for MRI. ▶K ♀C ▶? $$$

iohexol (*Omnipaque*): Iodinated, non-ionic, low osmolality IV and oral/body cavity contrast. ▶K ♀B ▶? $$$

iopamidol (*Isovue*): Iodinated, non-ionic, low osmolality IV contrast. ▶K ♀? ▶? $$

iothalamate (*Conray*): Iodinated, ionic, high osmolality IV contrast. ▶K ♀B ▶- $

ioversol (*Optiray*): Iodinated, non-ionic, low osmolality IV contrast. ▶K ♀B ▶? $$

ioxaglate (*Hexabrix*): Iodinated, ionic, low osmolality IV contrast. ▶K ♀B ▶- $$$

DERMATOLOGY

Acne Preparations

NOTE: Wash area prior to application. Wash hands before & after application; avoid eyes.

adapalene (*Differin*): apply qhs. [Trade only: gel 0.1%, 15,45 g.] ▶Bile ♀C ▶? $$

azelaic acid (*Azelex*): apply bid. [Trade only: cream 20%, 30g.] ▶K ♀B ▶? $$$

benzoyl peroxide (*Benzac, Desquam, Clearasil, Acetoxyl*): apply qd; increase to bid-tid if needed. [Generic: liquid 2.5,5,10%, bar 5,10%, mask 5%, lotion 5,5.5,10%, cream 5,10%, cleanser 10%, gel 2.5,4,5, 6,10,20%.] ▶LK ♀C ▶? $

clindamycin (*Cleocin T, Dalacin T*): apply bid. [Generic/Trade: gel 10 mg/ml 7.5,30g, lotion 10 mg/ml 60ml, solution 10mg/ml 30,60ml.] ▶L ♀B ▶- $

doxycycline (*Vibramycin, Doryx*): Acne vulgaris: 100 mg PO bid. [Generic only: tabs 50, caps 20, 50. Generic/Trade: Tabs 100, caps 50,100. Trade only: susp 25 mg/5 ml, syrup 50 mg/5ml (contains sulfites).] ▶LK ♀D ▶+ $$

erythromycin (*Eryderm, Erycette, Erygel, A/T/S, others*): apply bid. [Generic: solution 1.5% 60ml, 2% 60,120ml, pads 2%, gel 2% 30,60g, ointment 2% 25g.] ▶L ♀B ▶? $$

isotretinoin (*Accutane*): 0.5-2 mg/kg/day PO divided bid for 15-20 weeks. Typical target dose is 1mg/kg. Potent teratogen; extreme caution in women. Not for long-term use. [Trade only: caps 10,20,40.] ▶LK ♀X ▶- $$$$$

sodium sulfacetamide (*Klaron*): apply bid. [Trade only: lotion 10% 59ml.] ▶K ♀C ▶? $$

Sulfacet-R (sodium sulfacetamide & sulfur): apply 1-3 times daily. [Trade and generic: lotion (sodium sulfacetamide 10% & sulfur 5%) 25g.] ▶K ♀C ▶? $$

tazarotene (*Tazorac*): apply 0.1% gel qhs. [Trade only: gel 0.05% 30,100g, 0.1% 30, 100g.] ▶L ♀X ▶? $$$

tretinoin (*Retin-A, Renova, Retisol-A, Stievaa*): Apply qhs. [Generic/Trade: cream 0.025% 20,45g. Trade only: Retin-A cream 0.05% 20,45g, 0.1% 20,45g, gel 0.025% 15,45g, 0.01% 15,45g, liquid 0.05% 28ml. Trade only: Renova cream 0.05% 40,60g.] ▶? ♀C ▶? $$

Antibacterials (topical, see also acne preparations)

bacitracin: apply qd-tid. [Generic/Trade: ointment 500 units/g 1,15,30g.] ▶Not absorbed ♀C ▶? $

gentamicin (*Garamycin*): apply tid-qid. [Generic/Trade: ointment 0.1% 15,30g, cream 0.1% 15,30g.] ▶K ♀D ▶? $

mafenide (*Sulfamylon*): Apply qd-bid. [Trade only: cream 37,114,411g, 5% topical solution 50g packets.] ▶LK ♀C ▶? $$$

metronidazole (*Noritate, MetroGel, NidaGel*): Rosacea: apply bid. [Trade only: gel (MetroGel) 0.75% 29g, cream (Noritate) 1% 30g, lotion (MetroLotion) 0.75% 59ml.] ▶KL ♀B(- in 1st trimester) ▶- $$$

mupirocin (*Bactroban*): Impetigo/infected wounds: apply tid. Nasal MRSA eradication: 1 g divided between nostrils bid x 5 d. [Trade only: cream/ointment 2% 15,30g, nasal ointment 2% 1g single-use tubes (for MRSA eradication).] ▶Not absorbed ♀B ▶? $$

Neosporin cream (neomycin + polymyxin): apply qd-tid. [Trade only: neomycin 3.5 mg/g + polymyxin 10,000 units/g 15g and unit dose 0.94g.] ▶K ♀C ▶? $

Neosporin ointment (bacitracin + neomycin + polymyxin): apply qd-tid. [Generic/Trade: bacitracin 400units/g + neomycin 3.5 mg/g + polymyxin 5,000 units/g 2.4,9.6,14.2,15, 30g and unit dose 0.94g.] ▶K ♀C ▶? $

Polysporin (bacitracin + polymyxin): apply ointm't/aerosol/powder qd-tid. [Trade only: ointment 15,30g and unit dose 0.9g, powder 10g, aerosol 90g.] ▶K ♀C ▶? $

silver sulfadiazine (*Silvadene, Dermazin*): apply qd-bid. [Generic/Trade: cream 1% 20,50,85,400,1000g.] ▶LK ♀B ▶- $

Antifungals (topical)

amphotericin B (*Fungizone*): apply bid-qid. [Trade only: cream 3% 20g, lotion 3% 30ml, ointment 3% 20g.] ▶K ♀B ▶? $$$$

butenafine (*Mentax, Dr. Scholl's Athlete's Foot Cream*): apply qd-bid. [Trade only: cream 1% 15,30g.] ▶L ♀B ▶? $$$

ciclopirox (*Loprox, Penlac*): Cream, lotion: apply bid. Nail solution: apply daily to affected nails; apply over previous coat; remove with alcohol every 7 days. [Trade only: cream (Loprox) 1% 15,30,90g, lotion (Loprox) 1% 30,60ml, nail solution (Penlac) 8%.] ▶K ♀B ▶? $$

clotrimazole (*Lotrimin, Mycelex*): apply bid. [Generic/Trade: cream 1% 15,30,45,90g, solution 1% 10,30ml. Trade only: lotion 1% 30ml.] ▶L ♀B ▶? $

econazole (*Spectazole*): Tinea pedis, cruris, corporis, tinea versicolor: apply qd. Cutaneous candidiasis: apply bid. [Trade: cream 1% 15,30,85g.] ▶Not absorbed ♀C ▶? $$

haloprogin (*Halotex*): Tinea pedis, cruris, corporis, manuum, and versicolor: apply bid. [Trade only: cream 1% 15,30g, solution 1% 10,30ml.] ▶KL ♀B ▶? $$$

ketoconazole (*Nizoral*): Tinea/candidal infections: apply qd. Seborrheic dermatitis: apply cream qd-bid. Dandruff: apply 1% shampoo twice a week. Tinea versicolor: apply shampoo to affected area, leave on for 5 min, rinse. [Trade only: shampoo 1%,2%,120ml, cream 2% 15,30,60g.] ▶L ♀C ▶? $

miconazole (*Monistat-Derm, Micatin*): Tinea, candida: apply bid. [Generic: ointment 2% 29g, spray 2% 105ml, solution 2% 7.39,30ml. Generic/Trade: cream 2% 15,30,90g, powder 2% 90g, spray powder 2% 90,100g, spray liquid 2% 105,113ml.] ▶L ♀+ ▶? $

naftifine (*Naftin*): Tinea. apply qd (cream) or bid (gel). [Trade only: cream 1% 15,30,60g, gel 1% 20,40, 60g.] ▶LK ♀B ▶? $$

nystatin (*Mycostatin*): Candidiasis: apply bid/tid. [Generic/Trade: cream 100,000 units/g 15,30,240g, ointment 100,000 units/g 15,30g, powder 100,000 units/g 15g.] ▶Not absorbed ♀C ▶? $

oxiconazole (*Oxistat, Oxizole*): Tinea pedis, cruris, and corporis: apply qd-bid. Tinea versicolor (cream only): apply qd. [Trade only: cream 1% 15,30,60g, lotion 1% 30ml.] ▶? ♀B ▶? $$

terbinafine (*Lamisil*): Tinea: apply qd/bid. [Trade only: cream 1% 15,30g, gel 1% 5,15,30g, spray pump solution 1%.] ▶L ♀B ▶? $$$

tolnaftate (*Tinactin*): apply bid. [Generic/Trade: cream 1% 15,30g, solution 1% 10,15ml, powder 1% 45,90g, spray powder 1% 100,105,150g, spray liquid 1% 60,120ml. Trade only: gel 1% 15g.] ▶? ♀? ▶? $

Antiparasitics (topical)

A-200 (pyrethrins/piperonyl butoxide, R & C Shampoo): Lice: Apply shampoo, wash after 10 min. Reapply in 5-7 days. [Generic/Trade: shampoo (0.33% pyrethrins, 4% piperonyl butoxide) 60,120,240 ml.] ▶L ♀C ▶? $

crotamiton (*Eurax*): Scabies: apply cream/lotion topically from chin to feet, repeat in 24 hours, bathe 48 hours later. Pruritus: massage prn. [Trade only: cream 10% 60g, lotion 10% 60,480ml.] ▶? ♀C ▶? $$

lindane: Other drugs preferred. Scabies: apply 30-60ml of lotion, wash after 8-12h. Lice: 30-60 ml of shampoo, wash off after 4 min. Can cause seizures in epileptics or if overused/misused in children. Not for infants. [Generic/Trade: lotion 1% 30,60,480 ml, shampoo 1% 30,60,480ml.] ▶L ♀B ▶? $

malathion (*Ovide*): apply to dry hair, let dry naturally, wash off in 8-12 hrs. [Trade only: lotion 0.5% 59ml.] ▶? ♀B ▶? $$

permethrin (*Elimite, Acticin, Nix, Kwellada-P*): Scabies: apply cream from head (avoid mouth/ nose/eyes) to soles of feet & wash after 8-14h. 30 g is typical adult dose. Lice: Saturate hair and scalp with 1% rinse, wash after 10 min. Do not use in children < 2 months old. [Trade only: cream (Elimite, Acticin) 5% 60g. Trade/generic: liquid crème rinse (Nix) 1% 60ml.] ▶L ♀B ▶? $$

RID (pyrethrins/piperonyl butoxide): Lice: Apply shampoo/mousse, wash after 10 min. Reapply in 5-10 days. [Generic/Trade: shampoo 60,120,240 ml. Trade only: mousse 5.5 oz.] ▶L ♀C ▶? $

Antipsoriatics

acitretin (*Soriatane*): 25-50 mg PO qd. Avoid pregnancy during therapy and for 3 years after discontinuation. [Trade only: cap 10,25 mg.] ▶L ♀X ▶- $$$$$

anthralin (*Anthra-Derm, Drithocreme, Anthrascalp*): Apply qd. [Trade only: ointment 0.1% 42.5g, 0.25% 42.5g, 0.4% 60g, 0.5% 42.5g, 1% 42.5g, cream 0.1% 50g, 0.2% 50g, 0.25% 50g, 0.5% 50g. Generic/Trade: cream 1% 50g.] ▶? ♀C ▶- $$

calcipotriene (*Dovonex*): apply bid. [Trade only: ointment 0.005% 30,60,100g, cream 0.005% 30,60,100g, scalp solution 0.005% 60ml.] ▶L ♀C ▶? $$$

tazarotene (*Tazorac*): apply qhs. [Trade only: gel 0.05% 30,100g, 0.1% 30, 100g.] ▶Bile ♀X ▶? $$$

Antivirals (topical)

acyclovir (*Zovirax*): Herpes genitalis: apply q3h (6 times/d) for 7 days. [Trade only: ointment 5% 3,15g.] ▶K ♀C ▶? $$$

imiquimod (*Aldara*): Genital/perianal warts: apply 3 times weekly – put on at bedtime and wash off in 6-10 hours. [Trade only: cream 5% 250mg single use packets.] ▶Not absorbed ♀B ▶? $$$$

penciclovir (*Denavir*): Herpes labialis: apply cream q2h while awake x 4 days. [Trade only: cream 1% 2g tubes.] ▶Not absorbed ♀B ▶? $$$

podofilox (*Condylox, Condyline*): External genital warts (gel and solution) and perianal warts (gel only): apply bid for 3 consecutive days of a week and repeat for up to 4 wks. [Trade only: gel 0.5% 3.5g, solution 0.5% 3.5ml.] ▶? ♀C ▶? $$$

podophyllin (*Podocon-25, Podofin, Podofilm*): Warts: apply by physician. [Trade only: liquid 25% 15ml.] ▶? ♀- ▶- $$

Corticosteroid / Antimicrobial Combinations

Cortisporin (neomycin/polymyxin/hydrocortisone): apply bid/qid. [Generic/Trade: cream 7.5g, ointment 15g.] ▶LK ♀C ▶? $

Lotrisone (clotrimazole + betamethasone): apply bid. [Trade only: cream (clotrimazole 1% + betamethasone 0.05%) 15,45g.] ▶L ♀C ▶? $$$

Mycolog II (nystatin+trimacinolone): apply bid. [Generic/Trade: cream 15,30,60,120g, ointment 15,30,60,120g.] ▶L ♀C ▶? $

CORTICOSTEROIDS - TOPICAL* ♀C ▶?

Group / Agent	*Trade Name*	*Strength*	*Formulation*	*Frequency*
Group I (Most Potent)				
augmented beclomethasone dipropionate	*Diprolene*	0.05%	L, O, G	qd-bid
clobetasol propionate	*Temovate*	0.05%	C, O, G	bid
diflorasone diacetate	*Psorcon*	0.05%	S	qd-tid
flurandrenolide	*Cordran tape*	0.05%	O	bid
halobetasol propionate	*Ultravate*	0.05%	C, O	qd-bid
Group II				
amcinonide	*Cyclocort*	0.1%	O	bid-tid
betamethasone dipropionate	*Diprosone*	0.05%	O	qd-bid
"	*Maxivate*	0.05%	C,O	qd-bid
desoximetasone	*Topicort*	0.25%	C, O	bid
"	*Topicort*	0.05%	G	bid
diflorasone diacetate	*Florone, Maxiflor*	0.05%	O	qd-qid
fluocinonide	*Lidex*	0.05%	C, O, G	bid-qid
halcinonide	*Halog*	0.1%	C, O, S	bid-tid

Group III				
amcinonide	*Cyclocort*	0.1%	L	bid-tid
betamethasone benzoate	*Uticort*	0.025%	G, O	qd-bid
betamethasone dipropionate	*Diprosone*	0.05%	C	qd-bid
"	*Maxivate*	0.05%	O	qd-bid
betamethasone valerate	*Betatrex, Valisone*	0.1%	C	qd-bid
desoximetasone	*Topicort LP*	0.05%	C	bid
diflorasone diacetate	*Florone, Maxiflor*	0.05%	O	bid
fluticasone propionate	*Cutivate*	0.005%	O	qd
mometasone furoate	*Elocon*	0.1%	C, O	tid-qid
triamcinolone acetonide	*Aristocort, Aristocrt A, Kenalog*	0.5%	C, O	bid-qid
Group IV				
amcinonide	*Cyclocort*	0.1%	C	bid-tid
desoximetasone	*Topicort LP*	0.05%	C	bid-tid
fluocinilone acetonide	*Synalar HP*	0.2%	C	bid-qid
fluocinilone acetonide	*Synalar, Fluonide*	0.025%	O	bid-qid
fluandrenolide	*Cordran*	0.05%	O	bid-qid
halcinonide	*Halog*	0.025%	C, O	bid-tid
hydrocortisone valerate	*Westcort*	0.2%	O	bid-tid
mometasone furoate	*Elocon*	0.1%	C, L	tid-qid
triamcinolone acetonide	*Aristocort, Kenalog, Trymex*	0.1%	O	bid-qid
Group V				
betamethasone valerate	*Valisone, Betatrex*	0.1%	C, L	qd-bid
clocortolone pivalate	*Cloderm*	0.1%	C	qd-qid
desonide	*DesOwen, Tridesilon*	0.05%	O	bid-tid
flucinolone acetonide	*Synalar, Fluonide*	0.025%	C	bid-qid
flurandrenolide	*Cordran*	0.05%	C	bid-tid
"	*Cordran*	0.5%	L	bid-tid
"	*Cordran*	0.025%	O	bid-tid
"	*Cutivate*	0.05%	C	qd-bid
fluticasone	*Locoid*	0.1%	C, O, S	bid-tid
hydrocortisone butyrate	*Westcort*	0.2%	C	bid-tid
hydrocortisone valerate	*Dermatop*	0.1%	C	bid
prednicarbate	*Kenalog*	0.1%	C, L	tid-qid
triamcinolone acetonide	*Aristocort, Trymex*	0.1%	C	bid-qid
"	*Kenalog, Trymex*	0.025%	O	bid-qid
Group VI				
alclometasone dipropionate	*Aclovate*	0.05%	C, O	bid-tid
betamethasone valerate	*Valisone*	0.01%	C	qd-qid
desonide	*DesOwen*	0.05%	C, O, L	bid-tid
"	*Tridesilon*	0.05%	C	bid-qid
fluocinolone acetonide	*Synalar, Fluonid*	0.01%	C, S	bid-qid
triamcinolone acetonide	*Aristocort, Kenalog, Trymex*	0.025%	C	bid-qid
"	*Kenalog*	0.025%	L	bid-qid
Group VII (Least Potent)				
betamethasone valerate	*Celestone*	0.2%	C	qd-qid
hydrocortisone	*Hytone, others*	1, 2.5%	C, O, L	qd-qid

*__C-cream, G-gel, L-lotion, O-ointment, S-solution, T-tape__. Adapted from Habif TP, *Clinical Dermatology, 3rd ed.* Potency based on vasoconstrictive assays, which may not correlate with efficacy.

Hemorrhoid Care

Anusol Hemorrhoidal Ointment (pramoxine + zinc oxide + mineral oil): ointment/pads up to 5 times/day prn. [Trade only: ointment (Anusol Hemorrhoidal Ointment), pads (Fleet Pain Relief), aerosol foam (ProctoFoam NS).] ▶Not absorbed ♀+ ◗+ $

dibucaine (*Nupercainal*): apply cream/ointment tid/qid prn. [Generic/Trade: ointment 1% 30g.] ▶L ♀? ◗? $

hydrocortisone (*Anusol HC*): apply cream tid-qid prn or supp bid. [Generic/Trade: cream 1% (Anusol HC-1), 2.5% (Anusol HC), supp 25mg (Anusol HC).] ▶L ♀? ◗? $

Starch (Anusol Suppositories): 1 supp up to 6 times/day prn. [Trade only: supp (51% topical starch; soy bean oil, tocopheryl acetate).] ▶Not absorbed ♀+ ◗+ $

witch hazel (*Tucks*): Wipes to anus/perineum up to 6 times/day prn. [Generic/Trade: pads,gel.] ▶? ♀+ ◗+ $

Other Dermatologic Agents

alitretinoin (*Panretin*): Apply bid-qid to cutaneous Kaposi's lesions [Trade only: gel 60g.] ▶Not absorbed ♀D ◗- $$$$$

aminolevulinic acid (*Levulan Kerastick*): Apply solution to lesions on scalp or face; expose to blue illumination 14-18 h later. [Trade only: 20% solution single use ampules.] ▶Not absorbed ♀C ◗? ?

becaplermin (*Regranex*): Diabetic ulcers: apply gel qd. [Trade only: gel 0.01% 2,7.5,15g.] ▶Minimal absorption ♀C ◗? $$$$$

calamine: apply lotion tid-qid prn for poison ivy/oak or insect bite itching. [Generic: lotion 120, 240, 480ml.] ▶? ♀? ◗? $

capsaicin (*Zostrix, Zostrix-HP*): Arthritis, post-herpetic or diabetic neuralgia: apply cream up to tid-qid. [Generic/Trade: cream 0.025% 45,60g, 0.075% 30,60g, lotion 0.025% 59ml, 0.075% 59ml, gel 0.025% 15,30g, 0.05% 43g, roll-on 0.075% 60ml.] ▶? ♀? ◗? $

coal tar (*Polytar, Tegrin*): apply shampoo at least twice a week, or for psoriasis apply qd-qid. [Generic/Trade: shampoo, cream, ointment, gel, lotion, soap, oil.] ▶? ♀? ◗? $

doxepin (*Zonalon*): Pruritus: apply qid for up to 8 days. [Trade only: cream 5% 30,45g.] ▶L ♀B ◗- $

EMLA (lidocaine + prilocaine): Topical anesthesia: apply 2.5g cream or 1 disc to region at least 1 hour before procedure. Cover cream with an occlusive dressing. [Trade only: cream (2.5% lidocaine, 2.5% prilocaine) 5,30g, disc 1g.] ▶LK ♀B ◗? $$

finasteride (*Propecia*): Androgenetic alopecia in men: 1 mg PO qd. [Trade only: tab 1mg.] ▶L ♀X ◗- $$

fluorouracil (*5FU, Efudex, Fluoroplex*): Actinic keratoses: apply bid x 2-6 wks. Superficial basal cell carcinomas: apply 5% cream/solution bid. [Trade only: cream 5% 25g (Efudex), 1% 30g (Fluoroplex), solution 1% 30ml (Fluoroplex), 2% 10ml (Efudex), 5% 10ml (Efudex).] ▶L ♀X ◗- $$$$$

hydroquinone (*Eldopaque, Eldoquin, Esoterica, Lustra, Melanex, Solaquin*): Hyperpigmentation: apply to area bid. [Generic/Trade: cream 1.5,2,4%, lotion 2%, solution 3%, gel 4%.] ▶? ♀C ◗? $$$

lactic acid (*Lac-Hydrin*): apply lotion/cream bid. [Trade only: cream 12% 140,385g, lotion 12% 150,360ml.] ▶? ♀? ◗? $$

lidocaine (*Xylocaine, Lidoderm, Numby Stuff*): Apply prn. Postherpetic neuralgia: apply ≤3 patches for up to 12h in a 24h period. [Mouth/pharynx: spray 10%, ointment 5%, liquid 5%, solution 2,4%. Urethral jelly 2%. Patch (Lidoderm) 5%.] ▶LK ♀B ◗? $$

masoprocol (*Actinex*): Actinic keratoses: apply bid. [Trade only: cream 10% 30g.] ▶LK ♀B ▶? ?

minoxidil (*Rogaine, Rogaine Forte, Minoxidil for Men, Minox*): Androgenetic alopecia in men or women: 1 ml to dry scalp bid. [Trade only: solution 2%, 60ml, 5%, 60ml.] ▶K ♀C ▶- $$

oatmeal (*Aveeno*): Pruritus from poison ivy/oak, varicella: apply lotion qid prn. Also bath packets for tub. [Generic/Trade: lotion, packets.] ▶Not absorbed ♀? ▶? $

selenium sulfide (*Selsun, Exsel, Versel*): Dandruff, seborrheic dermatitis: apply 5-10 ml lotion/shampoo twice weekly x 2 weeks then less frequently, thereafter. Tinea versicolor: Apply 2.5% lotion/shampoo to affected area qd x 7 days. [Generic/Trade: lotion/shampoo 1% 120,210,240, 330ml, 2.5% 120ml.] ▶? ♀C ▶? $

Solag (mequinol/tretinoin): Apply to solar lentigines BID. [Trade only: soln 30ml (mequinol 2%/tretinoin 0.01%).] ▶Not absorbed ♀X ▶? ?

ENDOCRINE & METABOLIC

Androgens / Anabolic Steroids (See OB/GYN section for other hormones)

fluoxymesterone (*Halotestin*): 5-20 mg PO qd. [Trade: Tabs 2, 5 mg. Generic/Trade: Tabs 10 mg.] ▶L ♀X ▶? ©III $$

methyltestosterone (*Android, Methitest, Testred, Virilon, Metandren*): 10-40 mg PO qd. [Trade: Tabs 10 mg, Caps 10 mg. Generic/Trade: Tabs 25 mg.] ▶L ♀X ▶? ©III $$$

nandrolone decanoate (*Deca-Durabolin, Hybolin Decanoate*): 50-200 mg IM q week. [Generic/Trade: injection 100 mg/ml, 200 mg/ml. Trade only: injection 50 mg/ml.] ▶L ♀X ▶- ©III $$

testosterone (*Androderm, Androgel, Testoderm, Testoderm TTS, Depo-Testosterone, Depotest, Testro-L.A., Virilon IM, Delatestryl, Everone, Testro AQ*): Injectable enanthate or cypionate: 50-400 mg IM q2-4 wks. Transdermal - Androderm: 5 mg patch to nonscrotal skin hs; Testoderm TTS: one patch to arm/back/upper buttock qd. Testoderm: one patch to scrotal area qd. Androgel 1%: 1 gel pack (5 g) to shoulders/ upper arms/abdomen. [Trade only: patch 5 mg (Testoderm TTS). patch 4, 6 mg (Testoderm). patch 2.5, 5 mg (Androderm). gel 1%-2.5, 5 g (Androgel)] ▶L ♀X ▶? ©III $$$

Bisphosphonates

alendronate (*Fosamax*): Postmenopausal osteoporosis prevention (5 mg PO qd) & treatment (10 mg qd). Glucocorticoid-induced osteoporosis: 5-10 mg PO qd. Paget's disease: 40 mg PO qd x 6 mon. May cause esophagitis. [Trade: Tabs 5, 10, 40 mg.] ▶K ♀C ▶- $$$

etidronate (*Didronel*): Hypercalcemia: 7.5 mg/kg in 250 ml NS IV over ≥2h qd x 3d. Paget's disease: 5-10 mg/kg PO qd x 6 months or 11-20 mg/kg qd x 3 months. [Trade: Tabs 200, 400 mg.] ▶K ♀C ▶? $$$$

pamidronate (*Aredia*): Hypercalcemia: 60-90 mg IV single dose over 24h. Wait ≥7 days before considering retreatment. ▶K ♀C ▶? $$$$$

risedronate (*Actonel*): Paget's disease: 30 mg PO qd x 2 months. Osteoporosis prevention/treatment: 5 mg PO qd. May cause esophagitis. [Trade: Tabs 5, 30 mg.] ▶K ♀C ▶? $$$

tiludronate (*Skelid*): Paget's disease: 400 mg PO qd x 3 months. May cause esophagitis. [Trade: Tabs 200 mg.] ▶K ♀C ▶? $$$$$

Corticosteroids (See also dermatology, ophthalmology)

betamethasone (*Celestone, Beben*): 0.6-7.2 mg/day PO divided bid-qid; up to 9 mg/day IM. [Trade: Tabs 0.6 mg. syrup 0.6 mg/ 5 ml.] ▶L ♀C ▶- $$$$$

cortisone (*Cortone*): 25-300 mg PO qd. [Trade: Tabs 5, 10 mg. Generic/Trade: Tabs 25 mg.] ▶L ♀C ▶- $

dexamethasone (*Decadron, Dexasone, Dexone, Hexadrol*): 0.5-9 mg/day PO/IV/IM, divided bid-qid. [Generic/Trade: Tabs 0.25, 0.5, 0.75, 1.0, 1.5, 2, 4, 6 mg. elixir/ solution 0.5 mg/5ml. Trade only: oral solution 0.5 mg/ 0.5 ml. Decadron unipak (0.75 mg-12 tabs).] ▶L ♀C ▶- $

fludrocortisone (*Florinef*): Pure mineralocorticoid: 0.1 mg PO 3 times weekly to 0.2 mg PO qd. [Trade: Tabs 0.1 mg.] ▶L ♀C ▶? $

hydrocortisone (*Cortef, Solu-Cortef*): 100-500 mg IV/IM q2-10h as needed. 20-240 mg/day PO divided tid- qid. [Trade: Tabs 5, 10 mg. susp 10 mg/ 5 ml. Generic/Trade: Tabs 20 mg.] ▶L ♀C ▶- $

methylprednisolone (*Solu-Medrol, Medrol, Depo-Medrol*): Parenteral: dose varies, 10-250 mg IV/IM. Oral (Medrol): dose varies, 4-48 mg PO qd. Peds: 0.5-2 mg/kg PO/IV/IM. Medrol Dosepak tapers 24 to 0 mg PO over 7 days. IM/Joints (Depo-Medrol): dose varies, 4-120 mg IM q1-2 weeks. [Trade only: Tabs 2, 8, 16, 24, 32 mg. Generic/Trade: Tabs 4 mg. Medrol Dosepak (4 mg-21 tabs).] ▶L ♀C ▶- $$$

prednisolone (*Prelone, Pediapred*): 5-60 mg PO/IV/IM qd. [Generic/Trade: Tabs 5 mg. syrup 15 mg/ 5ml (Prelone; wild cherry flavor). Trade only: solution 5 mg/5ml (Pediapred; raspberry flavor).] ▶L ♀C ▶+ $$

prednisone (*Deltasone, Meticorten, Pred-Pak, Prednisone Intensol, Sterapred, Winpred, Metreton*): 1-2 mg/kg or 5-60 mg PO qd. [Generic/Trade: Tabs 1, 5, 10, 20, 50 mg. Trade only: Tabs 2.5 mg. Sterapred (5 mg-21& 48 tabs), Sterapred DS (10 mg-21,48, & 49 tabs) & Pred-Pak (5 mg- 45 & 79 tabs) taper packs. solution 5 mg/5 ml & 5 mg/ml (Intensol).] ▶L ♀C ▶+ $

triamcinolone (*Aristocort, Kenalog, Aristospan*): 4-48 mg PO/IM qd. [Generic/Trade: Tabs 4 mg. Trade only: injection 10 mg/ml, 25 mg/ml, 40 mg/ml.] ▶L ♀C ▶- $$$$

CORTICOSTEROIDS	*Approximate equivalent dose (mg)*	*Relative anti-inflammatory potency*	*Relative mineralocorticoid potency*	*Biologic Half-life (hours)*
betamethasone	0.6-0.75	20-30	0	36-54
cortisone	25	0.8	2	8-12
dexamethasone	0.75	20-30	0	36-54
hydrocortisone	20	1	2	8-12
methylprednisolone	4	5	0	18-36
prednisolone	5	4	1	18-36
prednisone	5	4	1	18-36
triamcinolone	4	5	0	18-36

Diabetes-Related - Sulfonylureas

glimepiride (*Amaryl*): Start 1-2 mg PO qd, usual 1-4 mg/day, max 8 mg/day. [Trade: Tabs 1, 2, 4 mg.] ▶LK ♀C ▶- $

glipizide (*Glucotrol, Glucotrol XL*): Start 5 mg PO qd, usual 10-20 mg/day, max 40 mg/day (divide bid if >15 mg/day). Extended release: Start 5 mg PO qd, usual 5-10 mg/day, max 20 mg/day. [Generic/Trade: Tabs 5, 10 mg. Trade only: extended release Tabs (Glucotrol XL) 2.5, 5, 10 mg.] ▶LK ♀C ▶? $

DIABETES NUMBERS*		Criteria for diagnosis of diabetes	Control	Hb A1c
Self-monitoring gluc. goals		(repeat to confirm on subsequent day)	Excellent	<7%
Preprandial	80-120 mg/dL	Fasting plasma glucose ≥126 mg/dL	Good	≤8%
Bedtime	100-140 mg/dL	Random plasma glucose ≥200 mg/dL	Take action	>8%

*http://ndep.nih.gov

glyburide (*Micronase, DiaBeta, Glynase PresTab, Euglucon*): Start 1.25-5 mg PO qd, usual 1.25-20 mg qd or divided bid, max 20 mg/day. Micronized tabs: Start 1.5-3 mg PO qd, usual 0.75-12 mg/day, max 12 mg/d. [Generic/Trade. Tabs 1.25, 2.5, 5 mg. micronized Tabs 1.5, 3, 6 mg.] ▶LK ♀B ▶? $

Diabetes-Related Agents - Other

acarbose (*Precose, Prandase*): Start 25 mg PO tid with meals; then gradually increase as tolerated to 50-100 mg tid. [Trade: Tabs 25, 50, 100 mg.] ▶Gut/K ♀B ▶- $$

dextrose (*Glutose, B-D Glucose, Insta-Glucose*): Hypoglycemia: 0.5-1 g/kg (1-2 ml/kg) up to 25 g (50ml) of 50% sol'n IV. Dilute before pediatric administration. [OTC/Trade only: chewable Tabs 5 g. gel 40%.] ▶L ♀C ▶? $

diazoxide (*Proglycem*): Hypoglycemia: 3-8 mg/kg/day divided q8-12h, max 10- 15 mg/kg/day. [Trade: susp 50 mg/ ml.] ▶L ♀C ▶- $$$$$

glucagon (*Glucagon, GlucaGen*): Hypoglycemia: 1 mg IV/IM/SC, onset 5-20 min. [Trade: injection 1 mg.] ▶LK ♀B ▶? $$$

glucose home testing (*Chemstrip bG, Dextrostix, Diascan,. Glucometer, Glucostix, Clinistix, Clinitest, Diastix, Tes-Tape*): [Blood: Chemstrip bG, Dextrostix, Diascan, Glucometer, Glucostix; Urine: Clinistix, Clinitest, Diastix, Tes-Tape] ▶None ♀+ ▶+ $$

Glucovance (glyburide + metformin): Start 1.25/250 mg PO qd or bid with meals as initial therapy; max 10/2000 mg/day. Or start 2.5/500 or 5/500 mg PO bid with meals as second-line therapy; max 20/2000 mg daily. May cause lactic acidosis. Hold prior to IV contrast agents and for 48 hours after. Avoid if ethanol abuse, CHF, renal or hepatic insufficiency. [Trade: tablets 1.25/250, 2.5/500, 5/500 mg] ▶KL ♀B ▶?

insulin (*Novolin, Novolog, Humulin, Humalog, Lantus*): Diabetes: 0.3-0.5 unit/kg/day SC in divided doses (Type I), and 1-1.5 unit/kg/day SC in divided doses (Type II), but doses vary. Humalog/Novolog- 0.5-1 unit/kg/day SC, but doses vary. Lantus- Start 10 units SC hs in insulin naïve patients, adjust to usual dose of 2-100 units/day. Severe hyperkalemia: 5-10 units regular insulin plus concurrent dextrose IV. Profound hyperglycemia (eg, DKA): 0.1 unit regular/kg IV bolus, infusion 100 units regular in 100 ml NS (1 unit/ml), at 0.1 units/kg/hr. 70 kg: 7 units/h (7 ml/h). Insulin lispro (Humalog): onset 0-15 min, peak ½- 1½ h, duration 3-4h. Insulin glargine (Lantus): slow, prolonged absorption. Regular: onset ½-1h, peak 2½-5h, duration 6-8h. NPH: onset 1-1½h, peak 4-12h, duration 24h. Mixtures of NPH and reg in 70/30 and 50/50 proportions. [Trade: injection NPH, regular, insulin lispro (Humalog), insulin lispro mix (Humalog Mix 75/25), insulin glargine (Lantus), insulin aspart (Novolog), regular and NPH mixtures (70/30 or 50/50).] ▶L ♀B/C ▶+ $$

metformin (*Glucophage, Glycon*): Start 500 mg PO qd/bid with meals, gradually increase prn to max 2550 mg/day. May cause lactic acidosis. Hold glucophage prior to IV contrast agents and for 48 hours after. Avoid if ethanol abuse, CHF, renal or hepatic insufficiency. [Trade: Tabs 500, 850, 1000 mg.] ▶K ♀B ▶? $$$

miglitol (*Glyset*): Start 25 mg PO tid with meals, maintenance 50-100 tid. [Trade: Tabs 25, 50, 100 mg.] ▶K ♀B ▶- $$$

pioglitazone (*Actos*): Start 15-30 mg PO qd, max 45 mg/day. Monitor LFTs. [Trade: Tabs 15, 30, 45 mg.] ▶L ♀C ▶- $$$

repaglinide (*Prandin, Gluconorm*): Start 0.5- 2 mg PO tid before meals, maintenance 0.5-4 mg tid-qid, max 16 mg/day. [Trade: Tabs 0.5, 1, 2 mg.] ▶L ♀C ◗? $$$

rosiglitazone (*Avandia*): Diabetes monotherapy or in combination with metformin or sulfonylurea: Start 4 mg PO qd or divided bid, max 8 mg/day monotherapy or in combination with metformin; max 4 mg/day in combination with sulfonylurea. Monitor LFTs q2 months for first year. [Trade: Tabs 2, 4, 8 mg.] ▶L ♀C ◗- $$$

Gout-Related

allopurinol (*Zyloprim, Purinol, Alloprin*): 200-300 mg PO qd/bid, max 800 md/day. [Generic/Trade: Tabs 100, 300 mg.] ▶K ♀C ◗? $

colchicine: Acute gouty arthritis: start 1- 1.2 mg PO, then 0.5- 1.2 mg PO q1-2h until pain relief or unacceptable side effects (i.e. diarrhea, GI upset); or 2 mg IV over 2-5 minutes, followed by 0.5 mg IV q6h. Max 8 mg/ day PO or 4 mg/day IV. Gout prophylaxis: 0.5- 1 mg PO qd- bid. [Generic/Trade: Tabs 0.5, 0.6 mg.] ▶L ♀D ◗+ $

probenecid (*Benemid, Benuryl*): Gout: 250 mg PO bid x 7 days, then 500 bid. Adjunct to penicillin injection: 1- 2 g PO. [Generic: Tabs 500 mg.] ▶KL ♀B ◗? $

Minerals

calcium acetate (*PhosLo*): Hyperphosphatemia: 2 tabs PO with each meal. [Trade only: tab 667mg (169 mg Ca).] ▶K ♀+ ◗? $

calcium carbonate (*Os-Cal, Os-Cal + D*): 250-2000 mg PO with meals bid-qid. [Generic/Trade: tab 650,667,1250,1500mg, chew tab 750,1250mg, cap 1250mg, susp 1250mg/5ml.] ▶K ♀+ ◗? $

calcium chloride: 500-1000 mg slow IV of 10% sol'n. [Generic: injectable 10% (1000mg/10ml) 10 ml ampules, vials, syringes.] ▶K ♀+ ◗? $

calcium gluconate: 2.25-14 mEq slow IV of 10% sol'n. 500-2000 mg PO bid-qid. [Generic: injectable 10% (1000mg/10ml, 4.65mEq/10ml) 10,50,100,200ml, tab 500,650,975,1000mg.] ▶K ♀+ ◗? $

ferrous gluconate (*Fergon*): 800-1600 mg ferrous gluconate PO tid. [Generic/Trade: tab 240,300,324,325.] ▶K ♀+ ◗+ $

ferrous polysaccharide (*Niferex*): 50-200 mg PO qd-tid. [Generic/Trade: (strength in terms of elemental mg iron): tab 50, cap 150, liquid 100mg/5ml.] ▶K ♀+ ◗+ $

ferrous sulfate (*Fer-in-Sol, FeoSol Tabs*): 500-1000 mg iron sulfate (100-200 mg elemental iron) PO divided tid. Liquid: Adults 5-10 ml tid, non-infant children 2.5-5 ml tid. Many other available formulations. [Generic/Trade: tab 324,325, liquid 220mg/5ml, drops 75mg/0.6ml.] ▶K ♀+ ◗+ $

fluoride (*Luride*): Adult dose: 10ml of topical rinse swish and spit qd. Peds daily dose based on fluoride content of drinking water (table). [Generic: chewable tab 0.5,1, tab 1, drops 0.125 mg/dropperful, 0.25 mg/dropperful, 0.5 mg/dropperful, lozenges 1, solution 0.2 mg/ml, gel 0.1%,0.5%,1.23%, rinse (sodium fluoride) 0.05,0.1,0.2%).] ▶K ♀? ◗? $

Peds qd dose is based on drinking water fluoride (shown in ppm)

Age (years)	*<0.3 ppm*	*0.3-0.6 ppm*	*>0.6 ppm*
0-0.5	none	none	none
0.5-3	0.25mg	none	none
3-6	0.5mg	0.25mg	none
6-16	1 mg	0.5 mg	none

iron dextran (*InFed, DexFerrum, Dexiron, Infufer*): 25-100 mg IM qd prn. Equations available to calculate IV dose for iron deficiency/blood loss. ▶KL ♀- ◗? $$$$

magnesium gluconate (*Almore, Magtrate, Maganate*): 500-1000 mg PO tid. [Generic: tab 500, liquid 54mg elem Mg/5ml.] ▶K ♀A ◗+ $

POTASSIUM, oral forms	Powders	Tablets/Capsules
Liquids	15 mEq/pack: *K-Lor*	6.7 mEq: *Kaon-Cl*
20 mEq/15 ml: *Cena-K, Kaochlor 10%, Kay Ciel, Klorvess, Kaon*	20 mEq/pack: *Kay Ciel, Kato, K-Lor, Klor-Con, Micro-K LS, Klorvess*	8 mEq: *Klor-Con 8, Slow-K, Micro-K*
40 mEq/15 ml: *Cena K, Kaon-Cl 20%*	25 mEq/pack: *K-Lyte-Cl, Klor-Con 25*	10 mEq: *Kaon-Cl 10, Klor-Con 10, Klotrix, K-Tab, K-Dur 10, Ten-K, Micro-K 10*
		20 mEq: *K-Dur 20*

magnesium oxide (*Mag-200, Mag-Ox 400*): 400-800 mg PO qd. [Generic/Trade: cap 140,250,400,420,500.] ▸K ♀A ▸+ $

magnesium sulfate: Hypomagnesemia: 1 g IM q6h q6h prn, or 2 g IV over 20 min. Peds: 25-50 mg/kg IV/IM. ▸K ♀A ▸+ $

phosphorous (*Neutra Phos, K-Phos*): 1 capsule or packet PO qid. 1-2 tabs PO tid/qid. Severe hypophosphatemia (eg, <1 mg/dl): 0.08-0.16 mmol/kg IV over 6h. [Generic/Trade: tab/cap/packet 250 mg (8 mmol) phosphorous.] ▸K ♀C ▸? $

potassium: IV infusion 10 mEq/h (diluted). 20-40 mEq PO qd-bid. [table] ▸K ♀C ▸? $

sodium ferric gluconate complex (*Ferrlecit*): 2 ml (25 mg elem iron) test dose diluted in 50 ml 0.9% sodium chloride IV over 60 minutes. If tolerated, then 10 ml (125 mg elem iron) diluted in 100 ml 0.9% sodium chloride IV over 1 hr. ▸KL ♀B ▸? $$$$$

Nutritionals

banana bag, rally pack: Alcoholic malnutrition (one formula): Add thiamine 100 mg + MgSO4 2g + IV multivitamins to one liter NS and infuse over 4h. "Banana bag" is jargon and not a valid drug order; specify individual components. ▸KL ♀+ ▸+ $

fat emulsion (*Intralipid, Liposyn*): dosage varies. ▸L ♀C ▸? $$$$$

formulas - infant (*Enfamil, Similac, Isomil, Nursoy, Prosobee, Soyalac, Alsoy*): Infant meals. [Milk-based (Enfamil, Silmilac, SMA) or soy-based (Isomil, Nursoy, Prosobee, Soyalac, Alsoy).] ▸L ♀+ ▸+ $

omega-3-fatty acids (*Promega, Max EPA*): 1-2 caps PO tid with meals. [Generic/Trade: cap 600,1000,1200mg (with varying ratios of EPA:DHA).] ▸L ♀- ▸? $

Thyroid Agents

levothyroxine (*T4, Synthroid, Levoxyl, Levothroid, L-thyroxine, Levotec, Eltroxin, Levo-T*): Start 50 mcg PO qd, increase by 25 mcg/day at 2-3 week intervals. Usual maintenance dose 100-200 mcg/day, max 300 mcg/d. [Generic/Trade: Tabs 25, 50, 75,100,125,150,200,300 mcg. Trade only: Tabs 88, 112, 137, 175 mcg.] ▸L ♀A ▸? $

liothyronine (*T3, Cytomel*): Start 25 mcg PO qd, max 100 mcg/day. [Trade only: Tabs 5 mcg. Generic/Trade: Tabs 25, 50 mcg.] ▸L ♀A ▸? $

methimazole (*Tapazole*): Start 5-20 mg PO tid, then adjust. [Trade: Tabs 5, 10 mg.] ▸L ♀D ▸+ $$$

propylthiouracil (*PTU*): Start 100 mg PO tid, then adjust. Thyroid storm: 200-300 mg PO qid, then adjust. [Generic: Tabs 50 mg.] ▸L ♀D (but preferred over methimazole) ▸+ $

Thyrolar (liotrix, levothyroxine (T4) and liothyronine (T3)): 1 PO qd, starting with small doses initially (¼-½ strength), then increase at 2 wk intervals. [Trade: Tabs T4/T3 12.5/3.1 (¼ strength), 25/6.25 (½ strength), 50/12.5 (#1), 100/25 (#2), 150/37.5 (#3) mcg.] ▸L ♀A ▸? $

Vitamins

ascorbic acid (*vitamin C*): 70-1000 mg PO qd. [Generic: tab 25,50,100,250,500,1000, chewable tab 100,250,500, time released tab 500, 1000,1500, time released cap 500, lozenge 60, liquid 35mg/0.6ml, sol'n 100mg/ml, syrup 500 mg/5ml.] ▶K ♀C ▶? $

calcitriol (*vitamin D, Rocaltrol, Calcijex*): 0.25-2 mcg PO qd. [Trade only: cap 0.25,0.5 mcg, oral soln 1mcg/ml.] ▶L ♀C ▶? $$

cyanocobalamin (*vitamin B12*): Deficiency states: 100-200 mcg IM q month or 25-250 mcg/d PO/intranasal. Some physicians give 1000 mcg IM periodically. [Generic: tab 25,50,100,250 mcg. Trade only: nasal gel 400 mcg/0.1 ml.] ▶K ♀C ▶+ $

dihydrotachysterol (*vitamin D, DHT*): 0.2-1.75 mg PO qd. [Generic: tab 0.125,0.2, 0.4, cap 0.125, solution 0.2 mg/ml.] ▶L ♀C ▶? $$

doxercalciferol (*Hecterol*): 10mcg PO three times a week. [Trade only: cap 2.5mcg.] ▶L ♀C ▶? $$$$

folic acid (*folate, Folvite*): 0.4-1 mg IV/IM/PO/SC qd. [Generic: tab 0.4,0.8,1mg.] ▶K ♀A ▶+ $

multivitamins (*MVI*): Dose varies with product. Tabs come with/without iron. [Many different brands/forms available (tab, cap, chewable tab, drops, liquid).] ▶LK ♀+ ▶+ $

niacin (*vitamin B3*): 10-500 mg PO qd. See cardiovascular section for lipid-lowering dose. [Generic: tab 25,50,100,250,500, timed release cap 125,250,300,400,500, liquid 50mg/5ml. Trade only: timed release tab (Niaspan) 375,500,750,1000, (Slo-Niacin) 250,500,750.] ▶K ♀C ▶? $

paricalcitol (*Zemplar*): CRF secondary hyperparathyroidism: 0.04-0.1 mcg/kg (2.8-7.0 mcg) IV 3 times/wk at dialysis. Max dose 0.24 mcg/kg (16.8 mcg). ▶L ♀C ▶? $$$$$

phytonadione (*vitamin K, Mephyton, AquaMephyton*): Single dose of 0.5-1 mg IM within 1h after birth. High INR due to warfarin: dose varies based on INR and clinical situation. [Trade only: tab 5.] ▶L ♀C ▶+ $

pyridoxine (*vitamin B6*): 10-200 mg PO qd. INH overdose: 1 g IV/IM q 30 min, total dose of 1 g for each gram of INH ingested. [Generic: tab 25,50,100, timed release tab 100.] ▶K ♀A ▶? $

riboflavin (*vitamin B2*): 5-25 mg PO qd. [Generic: tab 25,50,100.] ▶K ♀A ▶+ $

thiamine (*vitamin B1*): 10-100 mg IV/IM/PO qd. [Generic: tab 50,100,250,500, enteric coated tab 20.] ▶K ♀A ▶? $

tocopherol (*vitamin E*): RDA is 22 IU (natural, d-alpha-tochopherol) or 33 IU (synthetic, d,l-alpha-tochopherol). Antioxidant and "CHAOS" cardiac dose: 400-800 IU PO qd. [Generic: tab 200,400 IU, cap 73.5,100,147,165,200,330,400,500,600,1000 IU, drops 50 mg/ml.] ▶L ♀A ▶? $

Other Endocrine Agents

bromocriptine (*Parlodel*): Start 1.25- 2.5 mg PO qd, usual effective dose 2.5-15 mg/day, max 40 mg/day (hyperprolactinemia) or 20-30 mg/day, max 100 mg/day (acromegaly). [Generic/Trade: Tabs 2.5 mg. Caps 5 mg.] ▶L ♀B ▶- $$$$

cabergoline (*Dostinex*): Hyperprolactinemia: 0.25-1 mg PO twice/wk. [Trade: Tabs 0.5 mg.] ▶L ♀B ▶- $$$$$

calcitonin-salmon (*Calcimar, Miacalcin, Caltine*): Skin test before using: 1 unit intradermally and observe for local reaction. Osteoporosis: 100units SC/IM or 200 units nasal spray qd (alternate nostrils). Paget's disease: 50-100 units SC/IM qd. [Trade: nasal spray 200 units/ activation in 2 ml bottle (0.09 ml/dose).] ▶Plasma ♀C ▶? $$$

cosyntropin (*Cortrosyn, Synacthen*): Rapid screen for adrenocortical insufficiency: 0.25 mg (0.125 mg if <2 yo) IM/ IV over 2 min; measure serum cortisol before and 30-60 min after. ▶L ♀C ◗? $

desmopressin (*DDAVP, Stimate, Octostim*): Diabetes insipidus, enuresis: 10-40 mcg intranasally hs. [Trade only: Tabs 0.1, 0.2 mg. nasal solution 1.5 mg/ml (150 mcg/ spray). Generic/Trade: nasal solution 0.1 mg/ml (10 mcg/ spray). Note difference in concentration of nasal solutions.] ▶LK ♀B ◗? $$$$

growth hormone human (*Protropin, Genotropin, Norditropin, Nutropin, Humatrope, Serostim, Saizen*): Dosages vary by indication. ▶K ♀B/C ◗? $$$$$

oxifene (*Evista*): Osteoporosis prevention/treatment: 60 mg PO qd. [Trade: Tabs 60 mg.] ▶L ♀X ◗- $$$

sevelamer (*Renagel*): Hyperphosphatemia: 2-4 Caps tid with meals. [Trade: Caps 403 mg. Tabs 400, 800 mg.] ▶Not absorbed ♀C ◗? $$$$

sodium polystyrene sulfonate (*Kayexalate*): Hyperkalemia: 1 g/kg up to 15-60 g PO or 30-50 g retention enema (in sorbitol) q6h prn. Irrigate with tap water after enema to prevent necrosis. [Generic: susp 15 g/ 60 ml.] ▶Fecal excretion ♀? ◗? $$$$

spironolactone (*Aldactone*): Primary hyperaldosteronism, diagnosis: 400 mg/day PO x 4 days or 3-4 weeks. [Generic/Trade. Tabs 25, 50, 100 mg.] ▶LK ♀D ◗? $

tamoxifen (*Nolvadex, Tamofen, Tamone*): Breast cancer: 10-20 mg PO bid. [Generic/Trade: Tabs 10, 20 mg.] ▶L ♀D ◗- $$$$

vasopressin (*Pitressin*): Diabetes insipidus: 5-10 units IM/SC bid-qid prn. ▶LK ♀C ◗? $$$$$

ENT

Antihistamines - Nonsedating

fexofenadine (*Allegra*): 60mg PO bid or 180mg qd; 6-12 yo 30mg PO bid. [Trade: Tabs 30, 60, & 180mg; Caps 60mg.] ▶LK ♀C ◗? $$$

loratadine (*Claritin*): 10mg PO qd. [Trade: Tabs 10mg, fast-dissolve Reditabs 10mg; syrup 1mg/ml.] ▶LK ♀B ◗+ $$$

Antihistamines - Sedating

azatadine (*Optimine*): 1-2mg PO bid. [Trade: Tabs 1mg, scored.] ▶LK ♀B ◗- $$$

brompheniramine (*Dimetapp Allergy*): 4mg PO q4-6h. [OTC: Trade: Gel Caps 4mg; elixir 2mg/5ml; Generic/Trade: Tabs 4mg.] ▶LK ♀C ◗- $

cetirizine (*Zyrtec, Reactine*). 5-10mg PO qd for adults and children > 6 yo, 2.5mg/dose if 2-5 yo. [Trade: Tabs 5, 10 mg; syrup 5 mg/5ml.] ▶LK ♀B ◗- $$$

chlorpheniramine (*Chlor-Trimeton, Chlo-Amine, Aller-Chlor*): 4mg PO q4-6h; maximum 24mg/day. [OTC: Trade: Tabs chewable 2mg; Generic/Trade: Tabs 4mg; syrup 2mg/5ml. Generic/Trade: Tabs, Timed-release 8mg; Trade only: Tabs, Timed-release 12mg.] ▶LK ♀B ◗- $

clemastine (*Tavist*): 1.34mg PO bid, max 8.04mg/d. [OTC: Generic/Trade: Tabs 1.34 mg; Rx; Generic/Trade: Tabs 2.68mg; Trade only: Syrup 0.67mg/5ml.] ▶LK ♀B ◗- $

cyproheptadine (*Periactin*): Start 4mg PO tid, max 32mg/day. [Generic/Trade: Tabs 4mg (trade scored); syrup 2mg/5ml.] ▶LK ♀B ◗- $

dexchlorpheniramine maleate (*Polaramine*): 2mg PO q4-6h. Timed release tabs: 4 or 6mg PO at hs or q8-10h. [Trade: Tabs, Immediate Release 2mg; Syrup 2mg/5ml; Generic/Trade: Tabs, Timed Release: 4, 6mg.] ▶LK ♀? ◗- $$

ENT COMBINATIONS (selected)	Decon-gestant	Antihis-tamine	Anti-tussive	Typical Adult Doses
Actifed, Allerfrim	PS	TR	-	1 tab or 10 ml q4-6h
Allegra-D	PS	FE	-	1 tab q12h
Bromfenex	PS	BR		1 cap q12h
Claritin-D 12 hour	PS	LO	-	1 tab q12h
Claritin-D 24 hour	PS	LO	-	1 tab qd
Contac 12 Hour, Ornade	PP	CH	-	1 cap q12h
Deconamine	PS	CH	-	tab or 5-10 ml tid/qid
Deconamine SR	PS	CH	-	1 tab q12h
Deconsal II	PS	-	GU	1 tab q12h
Dimetapp	PP	BR	-	1 tab or 10 ml q4h*
Dimetapp Extentabs	PP	BR	-	1 tab q12h
Duratuss	PS	-	GU	1 tab q12h
Entex	PP, PE	-	GU	1 tab or 10 ml q6h
Entex LA	PP	-	GU	1 tab q12h
Entex PSE	PS	-	GU	1 tab q12h
Histussin D ©III	PS	-	HY	5 ml qid, prn
Histussin HC ©III	PE	CH	HY	10 ml q4h
Humibid DM	-	-	GU, DM	1-2 tabs q12h
Naldecon	PP	CH	-	1 tab bid/tid; 5 ml q4h
Phenergan/Dextromethorphn	-	PR	DM	5 ml q4-6h
Phenergan VC	PE	PR	-	5 ml q4-6h
Phenergan VC w/codeine©V	PE	PR	CO	5 ml q4-6h
Polyhistine	PT/PY/PH	-	-	10ml PO q4h
Robitussin AC ©V	-	-	GU, CO	10 ml q4h*
Robitussin CF	PP	-	GU, DM	10 ml q4h*
Robitussin DAC ©V	PS	-	GU, CO	10 ml q4h*
Robitussin DM	-	-	GU, DM	10 ml q4h*
Robitussin PE	PS	-	GU	10 ml q4h*
Rondec syrup	PS	CX	-	5 ml qid*
Rondec DM syrup	PS	CX	DM	5 ml qid*
Rondec Oral Infant Drops	PS	CX	-	0.25 to 1.0 ml qid†
Rondec DM Oral Infant drops	PS	CX	DM	0.25 to 1.0 ml qid†
Rynatan	PS	AZ	-	1 tab q12h
Symprex-D	PS	AC		1cap q4-6h up to 4/d
Triacin-C ©V	PS	TR	CO	10 ml q4-6h
Triaminic syrup	PP	CH	-	20 ml q4-6h‡
Triaminic DM syrup	PP	-	DM	20 ml q4h‡

AC=acrivastine; AZ=azatadine; BR=brompheniramine; CH=chlorpheniramine; CO=codeine; CX=carbinoxamine; DM=dextromethorphan; FE=fexofenadine; GU=guaifenesin; HY=hydrocodone; LO=loratadine; PE=phenylephrine; PH=pheniramine; PP=phenylpropanolamine; PR=promethazine; PS=pseudoephedrine; PT=phenyltolaxamine; PY=pyrilamine; TR=triprolidine

*5 ml/dose if 6-12 yo; 2.5 ml if 2-5yo. †1 ml/dose if 10-18 mo; ¾ ml if 7-9 mo; ½ ml if 4-6 mo; 1/4 ml if 1-3 months old. ‡10 ml/dose if 6-11 yo; 5 ml if 2-5 yo; 2.5 ml if 13-23 mo; 1.25 ml if 4-12 mo.

dimenhydrinate (*Dramamine, Gravol, Travel Tabs*): 50-100mg PO q4-6h. [OTC/Rx; Trade: Tabs 50mg; OTC: Trade only: Tabs, chewable 50mg; OTC: Generic/Trade: Liquid 12.5mg/4ml, OTC: Trade only: Liquid 12.5mg/5ml & Rx, Trade only: Liquid 15.62/5ml.] ▶LK ♀B ▶- $

diphenhydramine (*Benadryl, Allerdryl, Allernix*): 25-50mg IV/IM/PO q4-6h. Peds: 5mg/kg/day divided q4-6h. [OTC: Trade: Tabs 25, 50mg, Tabs, chewable 12.5mg; OTC & Rx: Generic/Trade: Caps 25, 50mg, softgel capsule 2 mg; OTC: Generic/ Trade: Liquid 6.25mg/5ml & 12.5mg/5ml.] ▶LK ♀B(- in 1st trimester) ▶- $

hydroxyzine (*Atarax* (hydrochloride salt), *Vistaril* (pamoate salt)): 25-100mg IM/PO qd-qid or prn. [Trade: Tabs 10, 25, 50, 100 mg; Caps 25, 50, 100 mg; syrup 10 mg/5 ml; susp 25 mg/5 ml.] ▶L ♀C ▶- $

promethazine (*Phenergan*): Adults: 12.5-25mg PO/IM/IV/PR qd-qid. Peds: 6.25-12.5mg PO/IM/IV/PR qd-qid. [Trade: Tabs 12.5mg, scored; Generic/Trade: Tabs 25, 50 mg; syrup 6.25mg/5ml; Trade only: syrup 25mg/5ml; Trade: Supp 12.5 & 25mg; Generic/Trade: Supp 50mg.] ▶LK ♀C ▶- $

Antitussives / Expectorants

benzonatate (*Tessalon Perles*): 100mg PO tid. Swallow whole. Do not chew; numbs mouth, possible choking hazard. [Generic: Caps, softgel 100mg; Trade: Perles 100mg.] ▶L ♀C ▶? $

dextromethorphan (*Benylin, Delsym, Vick's*): 10-20mg PO q4h or 30mg PO q6-8h. Sustained action liquid 60mg PO q12h. [OTC: Trade: Caps 30mg; lozenges 2.5, 5, 7.5, 15mg; liquid 3.5, 5, 7.5, 10, 12.5, 15mg/5ml; 10 & 15mg/15ml (Generic/Trade); Trade (Delsym): Sustained action liquid 30mg/5 ml.] ▶L ♀+ ▶? $

guaifenesin (*Robitussin, Humibid LA, Hytuss, Guiatuss,*): 100-400mg PO q4h; 600mg PO q12 (extended release). 100-200mg/dose if 6-11 yo; 50-100mg/dose if 2-5 yo. [OTC: Trade: Tabs 100mg; OTC & Rx; Trade: Tabs 200mg; Rx; Trade: Tabs 1200mg; Generic/Trade: Tabs, extended release 600 & 1200mg; OTC: Trade: Caps 200mg; Rx, Trade: Caps, sustained release 300mg; OTC & Rx; Trade: Syrup 100/5ml; OTC: Trade: Syrup 200mg/5 ml.] ▶L ♀C ▶? $

Hycodan (hydrocodone/homatropine): 1 tab or 5 mL PO q4-6h. [Trade: Tabs 5/1.5; Generic/Trade; Syrup 5/1.5 per 5ml.] ▶L ♀C ▶- ©III $

Decongestants (See Nasal Preparations for topical nasal spray decongestants)

phenylpropanolamine (*Propagest*): 25mg PO q4h. Sustained release: 75mg PO q12h. [OTC; Generic/Trade: Tabs 25mg; Generic only: Tabs 50mg; Trade: Tabs, extended release 75mg; Generic only: Caps, extended release 75mg.] ▶L ♀C ▶- $

pseudoephedrine (*Sudafed, Sudafed 12 Hour, Efidac/24, PediaCare Infants' Decongestant, Triaminic Oral Infant Drops*): Adult: 60mg PO q4-6h; Peds: 30mg/dose if 6-12 yo, 15mg/dose if 2-5 yo. Ext rel tabs: 120mg PO bid or 240mg PO qd. Pediacare Infant Drops & Triaminic Infant Drops (7.5mg/0.8ml): 2-3 yo: 1.6ml PO q4-6h; 12-23 mo: 1.2ml PO q4-6h; 4-11 mo: 0.8ml PO q4-6h; 0-3 mo: 0.4ml PO q4-6h; maximum 4 doses/day. [OTC: Generic/Trade: Tabs 30, 60 mg; chewable Tabs 15mg. Trade only: Tabs, extended release 120, 240mg; Trade only: Liquid, 15mg/5ml; Generic/Trade: Liquid, 30mg/5ml; Trade only: infant drops 7.5mg/0.8ml.] ▶L ♀C ▶+ $

Ear Preparations

Auralgan (benzocaine/antipyrine): 2-4 drops in ear(s) tid/qid prn. [Generic/Trade: Otic sol'n 10 & 15ml.] ▶Not absorbed ♀C ▶? $

carbamide peroxide (*Debrox, Murine Ear*): 5-10 drops in ear(s) bid. [OTC: Trade: Otic sol'n 6.5% ,15 or 30ml bottle.] ▶Not absorbed ♀? ▶? $

Cipro HC Otic (ciprofloxacin/hydrocortisone): ≥1 yo to adult: 3 drops in ear(s) bid x 7 days. [Trade: Otic susp 10ml bottle.] ▶Not absorbed ♀C ▶- $$$

Cortisporin otic (hydrocortisone/polymyxin/neomycin): 4 drops in ear(s) tid/qid of sol'n or susp (use susp if TM perforation). Peds: Otitis externa: 3 drops in ear(s) tid-qid. [Generic/Trade: Otic sol'n or susp 7.5 & 10ml.] ▶Not absorbed ♀? ▶? $$

Cortisporin TC (hydrocortisone/neomycin/thonzium/colistin): 4-5 drops in ear(s) tid-qid. [Trade: Otic susp, 10ml.] ▶Not absorbed ♀? ▶? $$

Domeboro Otic (acetic acid/aluminum acetate): 4-6 drops in ear(s) q2-3h; Peds:2-3 drops in ear(s) q3-4h. [Generic/Trade: Otic sol'n 60ml bottle.] ▶Not absorbed ♀? ▶? $

ofloxacin (*Floxin Otic*): >12 yo: 10 drops in ear(s) bid; 1-12 yo: 5 drops in ear(s) bid. [Trade: Otic sol'n 0.3% 5 ml bottle.] ▶Not absorbed ♀C ▶- $$

Otobiotic (hydrocortisone/polymyxin B): 3-4 drops in ear(s) tid-qid. [Trade: Otic sol'n 0.5%, 1 ml.] ▶Not absorbed ♀? ▶? $

Pediotic (hydrocortisone/polymyxin/neomycin): 3-4 drops in ear(s) tid/qid. [Trade: Otic susp 7.5ml.] ▶Not absorbed ♀? ▶? $$

Swim-Ear (isopropyl alcohol 95%/anhydrous glycerins 5%): 4-5 drops in ears after swimming. [OTC: Trade: Otic sol'n 30ml bottle.] ▶Not absorbed ♀? ▶? $

triethanolamine (*Cerumenex*): Fill ear canal x 15-30 mins to loosen cerumen, then flush. [Trade: Otic sol'n 6 & 12ml bottle with dropper.] ▶Not absorbed ♀C ▶- $$

VoSol otic (acetic acid/propylene glycol): 5 drops in ear(s) tid/qid; Peds > 3 yo: 3-4 drops in ear(s) tid/qid. [Generic/Trade: Otic sol'n 2% 15 & 30ml bottle.] ▶Not absorbed ♀? ▶? $

Mouth & Lip Preparations

amlexanox (*Aphthasol*): Aphthous ulcers: Apply ¼ inch paste qid after oral hygiene. [Trade: Oral paste 5%, 5g tube.] ▶LK ♀B ▶? $

chlorhexidine gluconate (*Peridex, Periogard*): Rinse with 15ml of undiluted sol'n for 30 seconds twice daily. Not intended for ingestion; expectorate after rinsing. [Trade: Oral rinse 0.12% 473-480ml bottles.] ▶Fecal excretion ♀B ▶? $

clotrimazole (*Mycelex*): Oral troches dissolved slowly in mouth 5 times/day x 14 days. [Trade: Oral troches 10mg.] ▶L ♀C ▶? $$$

lidocaine viscous (*Xylocaine*): Mouth or lip pain in adults only: 15ml topically or swish & spit q3h. [Generic/Trade: sol'n 2%, 20,50,100,450ml bottles.] ▶LK ♀B ▶+ $

magic mouthwash (*Benadryl/Mylanta or Maalox/Carafate*): 5ml PO swish and spit or swish and swallow tid before meals and prn. [Compounded susp. A standard receipe would be 30ml diphenhydramine elixir/60ml Mylanta or Maalox/4g Carafate.] ▶LK ♀B(- in 1st trimester) ▶- $$$

nystatin (*Mycostatin*): Thrush: 5ml PO swish & swallow qid. Infants: 2ml/dose with 1ml placed in each cheek. [Generic/Trade: Susp 100,000 units/ml 60 & 480ml bottle, Trade: oral lozenges (Pastilles) 200,000 units.] ▶Not absorbed ♀C ▶? $$

penciclovir (*Denavir*): Herpes labialis (cold sores): apply cream q2h while awake x 4d. Start at first sign of symptoms. [Trade: Cream 1%, 1.5g tube.] ▶Not absorbed ♀B ▶- $

triamcinolone acetonide (*Kenalog in Orabase*): Apply the paste 2-3 times per day. The best times are usually after a meal and at bedtime. [Generic/Trade: 0.1% oral paste 5g tubes] ▶L ♀C ▶? $

Nasal Preparations

azelastine (*Astelin*): Allergic rhinitis: 2 sprays in each nostril bid. [Trade: Nasal spray, 100 sprays/bottle (17ml).] ▶L ♀C ▶? $$

beclomethasone (*Vancenase, Vancenase AQ, Vancenase AQ Double Strength, Beconase, Beconase AQ*): Vancenase, Beconase: 1 spray bid-qid. [42mcg/spray]. Vancenase AQ, Beconase AQ: 1-2 spray(s) in each nostril bid. [42mcg/spray]. Vancenase AQ Double Strength [84mcg/spray]: 1-2 spray(s) in each nostril qd. [Trade: Nasal inhalation aerosol (Beconase, Vancenase) 42mcg/spray. Nasal aqueous susp (Beconase AQ, Vancenase AQ) 42mcg/spray. Nasal aqueous susp double strength (Vancenase AQ Double Strength) 84mcg/spray.] ▶L ♀C ▶? $$

budesonide (*Rhinocort, Rhinocort Aqua*): 2 sprays in each nostril bid or 4 sprays qd (Rhinocort); 1-4 sprays/nostril qd (Rhinocort Aqua). [Trade: (Rhinocort): Nasal inhaler 200 sprays/bottle; (Rhinocort Aqua) 32mcg/spray: 60 and 120 sprays/bottle, 64mcg/spray: 120 sprays/bottle.] ▶L ♀C ▶? $$

flunisolide (*Nasalide, Nasarel, Rhinalar*): Start 2 sprays in each nostril bid, max 8 sprays/day. [Trade: Nasal sol'n 0.025%, 200 sprays/bottle (25ml). Nasalide with pump unit; Nasarel with meter pump & nasal adapter.] ▶L ♀C ▶? $$

fluticasone (*Flonase*): 2 sprays in each nostril qd. [Trade: Nasal spray 0.05%, 120 sprays/bottle (16ml).] ▶L ♀C ▶? $$$

ipratropium nasal spray (*Atrovent Nasal Spray 0.03%, 0.06%*): 2 sprays in each nostril bid-qid. [Trade: Nasal spray 0.03%, 345 sprays/bottle (30ml) & 0.06%, 165 sprays/bottle (15ml).] ▶Lung ♀B ▶? $$

mometasone (*Nasonex*): Adult: 2 sprays in each nostril qd; Peds 3-11 yo: one spray in each nostril qd. [Trade: Nasal spray, 120 sprays/bottle (17ml).] ▶L ♀C ▶? $$$

oxymetazoline (*Afrin, Dristan 12 Hr Nasal, Nostrilla*): 2-3 drops/sprays in each nostril bid X 3 days. [OTC: Generic/Trade: Nasal spray 0.05%, 15 & 30ml bottles; nose drops 0.025% & 0.05%, 20ml w/dropper.] ▶L ♀C ▶? $

phenylephrine (*Neo-Synephrine, Sinex, Nostril*): 2-3 sprays/drops in each nostril q4h prn X 3 days. [OTC: Trade: Nasal drops 0.125, 0.16%; Generic/Trade: Nasal spray/drops 0.25, 0.5, 1%.] ▶L ♀C ▶? $

saline nasal spray (*SeaMist, Pretz, NaSal, Ocean*): 1-3 sprays or drops prn. [Generic/Trade: Nasal spray 0.4, 0.5, 0.6, 0.65, 0.75%; nasal drops 0.4, 0.65, & 0.75%.] ▶Not metabolized ♀A ▶+ $

triamcinolone (*Nasacort, Nasacort AQ*): Nasacort: 2 sprays in each nostril qd/bid, max 8 sprays/day. Nasacort AQ: 2 sprays in each nostril qd. [Trade: Nasal inhaler 100 sprays/bottle, 10g (Nasacort); nasal pump 120 sprays/bottle, 16.5g (Nasacort AQ).] ▶L ♀C ▶- $$

triamcinolone acetonide (*Tri-Nasal*): 2-4 sprays in each nostril qd. [Trade: 50mcg/spray, 120 sprays/bottle (15ml).] ▶L ♀C ▶? $$

GASTROENTEROLOGY

Antidiarrheals

attapulgite (*Kaopectate, Diasorb, Donnagel*): 1200-1500 mg PO after each loose BM; max 9000 mg/day. Dose 600-1500 mg if 6-12 yo, 300-750 mg if 3-6 yo. [Generic/Trade: liquid 600mg&750mg/15ml (Donnagel, Kaopectate), 750mg/5ml (Diasorb), tab 750, chewable tab 300,600,750.] ▶Not absorbed ♀+ ▶+ $

bismuth subsalicylate (*Pepto-Bismol*): 2 tabs or 30 ml PO q 30min-1h up to 8 doses/ 24h. Peds: 10 ml or 2/3 tab if 6-9 yo, 5 ml or 1/3 tab if 3-6 yo. Risk of Reye's syndrome in children. [Generic/Trade: chewable tab 262, susp 262 & 524mg/15ml. Generic only: susp 130 mg/15ml. Trade only: caplets 262mg.] ▶K ♀D ◗? $

Lomotil (diphenoxylate + atropine): 2 tabs or 10 ml PO qid. [Generic/Trade: solution 2.5mg diphenoxylate + 0.025 mg atropine per 5ml, tab 2.5mg diphenoxylate + 0.025 mg atropine per tablet.] ▶L ♀C ◗- ©V ?

loperamide (*Imodium, Imodium AD, Loperacap*): 4 mg PO initially, then 2 mg PO after each unformed stool to a maximum of 16 mg/day. Peds: 2 mg PO tid if >30 kg, 2 mg bid if 20-30 kg, 1 mg tid if 13-20 kg. [Generic/Trade: cap 2, tab 2, liquid 1 mg/5ml.] ▶L ♀B ◗+ $

Antiemetics - 5-HT3 Receptor Antagonists

dolasetron (*Anzemet*): Nausea with chemo: 1.8 mg/kg up to 100 mg IV/PO single dose. Post-op nausea: 12.5 mg IV in adults and 0.35 mg/kg IV in children as single dose. Alternative for prevention 100 mg (adults) or 1.2 mg/kg (children) PO 2 hours before surgery. [Trade only: tab 50,100.] ▶LK ♀B ◗? $$$

granisetron (*Kytril*): Nausea with chemo: 10 mcg/kg IV over 5 minutes, 30 minutes prior to chemo. Oral: 1 mg PO bid x 1 day only. Radiation induced N/V: 2 mg PO 1 hr before first irradiation fraction of each day. [Trade only: tab 1mg.] ▶L ♀B ◗? $$$

ondansetron (*Zofran*): Nausea with chemo: 32 mg IV over 15 min, or 0.15 mg/kg doses 30 min prior to chemo and repeated at 4 & 8 hrs after first dose. Oral dose if ≥12 yo: 8 mg PO bid. If 4-11 yo: 4 mg PO tid. Post-op nausea: 4 mg IV/IM over 2-5 min or 16 mg PO 1 hr before anesthesia. Prevention radiation N/V: 8 mg PO tid. [Trade only: tab 4,8,24 orally disintegrating tab 4, 8, solution 4mg/5ml.] ▶L ♀B ◗? $$$

Antiemetics - Other

dimenhydrinate (*Dramamine, Marmine*): 50-100 mg PO/IM/IV q4-6h prn. [Generic/Trade: tab/cap 50, liquid 12.5mg/4ml. Trade only: chewable tab 50, liquid 12.5 & 15.62mg/5ml.] ▶LK ♀B ◗- $

doxylamine (*Unisom Nighttime Sleep Aid, others*): 12.5 mg PO BID; often used in combination with pyridoxine. ▶L ♀A ◗? $

dronabinol (*Marinol*): Nausea with chemo: 5mg/m^2 1-3 h before chemo then 5mg/m^2/ dose q2-4h after chemo for 4-6 doses/day. AIDS anorexia: Initially 2.5 mg PO bid before lunch and dinner. [Trade only: cap 2.5,5,10.] ▶L ♀C ◗- ©III $$$$$

droperidol (*Inapsine*): 0.625-2.5 mg IV or 2.5-10 mg IM. ▶L ♀C ◗? $

metoclopramide (*Reglan, Maxeran*): 10 mg IV/IM q2-3h prn. 10-15 mg PO qid, 30 min before meals and hs. [Generic/Trade: tabs 5,10, liquid 5mg/5ml.] ▶K ♀B ◗+ $$

phosphorated carbohydrates (*Emetrol*): 15-30 ml PO q15min prn, max 5 doses. Peds: 5-10 ml. [Generic/Trade: Solution containing dextrose and fructose.] ▶L ♀A ◗+ $

prochlorperazine (*Compazine, Stemetil*): 5-10 mg IV over at least 2 min. 5-10 mg PO/IM tid/qid. 25 mg PR q12h. Sustained release: 15 mg PO qam or 10 mg PO q12h. Peds: 0.1 mg/kg/dose PO/PR tid-qid or 0.1-0.15 mg/kg/dose IM tid-qid. [Generic/Trade: tabs 5,10,25, supp 25. Trade only: extended release (Compazine Spansules) 10,15,30, supp 2.5,5, liquid 5mg/5ml.] ▶LK ♀C ◗? $

promethazine (*Phenergan*): Adults: 12.5-25 mg PO/IM/PR q4-6h. Peds: 0.25-0.5 mg/kg PO/IM/PR q4-6h. Unapproved IV use common. [Generic/Trade: tab 25,50, syrup 6.25 mg/5ml, supp 50. Trade only: tab 12.5, syrup 25mg/5ml, supp 12.5,25.] ▶LK ♀C ◗- $

scopolamine (*Transderm Scop, Transderm-V*): Motion sickness: Apply 1 disc (1.5 mg) behind ear 4h prior to event; replace q3 days. [Trade only: topical disc 1.5mg/72h, box of 4.] ▶L ♀C ◗+ $

trimethobenzamide (*Tigan*): 250 mg PO q6-8h, 200 mg IM/PR q6-8h. Peds: 100-200 mg/dose PO/PR q6-8h if 13.6-40.9 kg; 100 mg PR q6-8h if <13.6kg (not newborns). [Generic/Trade: caps 100,250, supp 100,200.] ▶LK ♀C but + ◗? $

Antiulcer - Antacids

aluminum hydroxide (*Alternagel, Amphojel, Alu-tab*): 5-10 ml or 1-2 tabs PO up to 6 times daily. Constipating. [Generic/Trade: tabs 300,475,500,600, susp 320,450,600, 675 mg/5ml.] ▶K ♀+ (? 1st trimester) ◗? $

calcium carbonate (*Tums, Mylanta Children's, Titralac, Rolaids Calcium Rich, Viactiv*): 1000-3000 mg PO q2h prn, max 8000mg/d. [Generic/Trade: tabs 350,400,420,500, 550,650,750, 850,1000mg, susp 400,1250mg/5ml.] ▶K ♀+ (? 1st trimester) ◗? $

Maalox (aluminum & magnesium hydroxide): 10-20 ml or 1-4 tab PO prn. [Generic/Trade: Chewable tabs, susp.] ▶K ♀+ (? 1st trimester) ◗? $

magaldrate (*Riopan*): 5-10 ml PO prn. [Generic/Trade: susp 540mg/5ml. (Riopan Plus avail as susp 540, 1080mg/5ml, chew tab 480, 1080).] ▶K ♀+ (? 1st trimester) ◗? $

Mylanta susp (aluminum & magnesium hydroxide + simethicone): 2-4 tab or 10-45 ml PO prn. [Generic/Trade: Liquid, double strength liquid, tab, double strength tab.] ▶K ♀+ (? 1st trimester) ◗? $

Antiulcer - H2 Antagonists

cimetidine (*Tagamet, Tagamet HB, Gaviscon Prevent, Peptol*): 300 mg IV/IM/PO q6-8h, 400 mg PO bid, or 400-800 mg PO qhs. Continuous IV infusion 37.5-50 mg/h (900-1200 mg/day). [Generic/Trade: tab 200,300,400,800, liquid 300mg/5ml. Trade only: tab 100 (OTC, Tagamet HB).] ▶LK ♀B ◗+ $$$

famotidine (*Pepcid, Pepcid AC*): 20 mg IV q12h. 20-40 mg PO qhs, or 20 mg PO bid. [Trade only: tabs 10 (OTC, Pepcid AC Acid Controller),20,40, susp 40mg/5ml.] ▶LK ♀B ◗? $$$$

nizatadine (*Axid*): 150-300 mg PO qhs, or 150 mg PO bid. [Trade only: tabs 75 (OTC, Axid AR), cap 150,300.] ▶K ♀C ◗? $$$$

ranitidine (*Zantac, Zantac 75, Peptic Relief*): 150 mg PO bid or 300 qhs. 50 mg IV/IM q8h, or continuous infusion 6.25 mg/h (150 mg/d). [Generic/Trade: tabs 150,300, syrup 75mg/5ml. Trade only: tab 75 (OTC, Zantac 75), effervescent tab 150, caps 150,300, granules 150.] ▶K ♀B ◗? $$$

Antiulcer - Helicobacter pylori Treatment

Helidac (bismuth subsalicylate + metronidazole + tetracycline): 1 dose PO qid for 2 weeks. To be given with an H2 antagonist. [Trade only: Each dose: bismuth subsalicylate 524 (2x262 mg) + metronidazole 250 mg + tetracycline 500 mg.] ▶LK ♀D ◗- $$

PrevPac (lansoprazole + amoxicillin + clarithromycin): 1 dose PO bid x 14 days. [Trade only: lansoprazole 30 mg + amoxicillin 1 g (2x500mg), clarithromycin 500 mg.] ▶LK ♀C ◗? $$$$$

Tritec (ranitidine bismuth citrate): 400 mg PO bid x 4 weeks in conjunction with clarithromycin 500 mg PO tid for first 2 weeks. [Trade only: tab 400.] ▶K ♀C ◗? $$$

HELICOBACTER PYLORI TREATMENT

*Regimen**	*Dosing*	*Eradication*
lansoprazole, and clarithromycin, and amoxicillin *(PrevPac)*	30 mg PO bid x 14 days 500 mg PO bid x 14 days 1g PO bid x 14 days EQUALS 1 *Prevpac* dose PO bid x 2 wks	86%
omeprazole, and clarithromycin, and amoxicillin	20 mg PO bid x 14 days 500 mg PO bid x 14 days 1 g PO bid x 14 days	80-86%
lansoprazole, or omeprazole, and clarithromycin, and metronidazole	30 mg PO bid x 14 days or 20 mg PO bid x 14 days 500 mg PO bid x 14 days 500 mg PO bid x 14 days	≥ 80%
lansoprazole, or omeprazole, and BSS, and metronidazole and tetracycline	30 mg PO qd x 14 days or 20 mg PO qd x 14 days 525mg PO qid x 14 days 500 mg PO tid x 14 days 500 mg PO qid x 14 days	83-95%
famotidine, or ranitidine, or nizatidine, and BSS, and metronidazole, and tetracycline**	40 mg/d PO qd/bid x 28 days or 300 mg/day PO qd/bid x 28 days or 300 mg/day PO qd/bid x 28 days 525 mg PO qid x initial14 days 250 mg PO qid x initial14 days 500 mg PO qid x initial14 days	≥ 80%
RBS, and clarithromycin, and amoxicillin, or metronidazole, or tetracycline	400 mg PO bid x 14 days 500 mg PO bid x 14 days 1 g PO bid x 14 days or 500 mg PO bid x 14 days or 500 mg PO bid x 14 days	≥ 80%

**American College of Gastroenterology Guidelines (Am J Gastroenterol 1998; 93:2330).*
BSS=bismuth subsalicylate (Pepto-Bismol) RBS=ranitidine bismuth citrate (Tritec)
***BSS,metronidazole, tetracycline available as Helidac.*

Antiulcer - Other

dicyclomine (*Bentyl, Bentylol*): 10-20 mg PO/IM qid up to 40 mg PO qid. [Generic/Trade: tab 20, cap 10, syrup 10mg/5ml. Generic only: cap 20.] ▶LK ♀B ▶- $$

Donnatal (phenobarbital/atropine/hyoscyamine/scopolamine): 1-2 tabs/caps or 5-10 ml PO tid/qid. 1 extended release tablet PO q8-12h. [Generic/Trade: 16.2/0.02/0.1/0.0065 mg in each tab, cap or 5ml. Each extended release tablet has 48.6/0.0582/0.3111/0.0195 mg.] ▶LK ♀C ▶- $

GI cocktail (eg, "green goddess"): Acute GI upset: mixture of Maalox/Mylanta 30 ml + viscous lidocaine (2%) 10 ml + Donnatal 10 ml administered PO in a single dose. ▶LK ♀See individual ▶See individual $

hyoscyamine (*Levsin*): 0.125-0.25 mg PO/SL tid-qid. Sustained release: 0.375-0.75 mg PO q12h. [Generic/Trade: tab 0.125,0.15, SL tab 0.125, solution 0.125 mg/ml. Trade only: extended release tab/cap 0.375, elixir 0.125mg/5ml.] ▶LK ♀C ▶- $

misoprostol (*Cytotec*): Prevention of NSAID-induced gastric ulcers: Start 100 mcg PO bid, then titrate as tolerated up to 200 mcg PO qid. Abortifacient. Diarrhea in 13-40%, abdominal pain in 7-20%. [Trade only: tab 100,200 mcg.] ▶LK ♀X ▶- $$$$

propantheline (*Pro-Banthine*): 7.5-15 mg PO 30 min ac & qhs. [Generic/Trade: tab 15, Trade only: tab 7.5.] ▶LK ♀C ◗- $$$

simethicone (*Mylicon, Gas-X, Phazyme*): 40-160 mg PO qid prn. Infants: 20 mg PO qid prn [Generic/Trade: tab 60,95, chewable tab 40,80,125, cap 125, drops 40mg/0.6ml.] ▶Not absorbed ♀C but + ◗? $

sucralfate (*Carafate*): 1 g PO 1h before meals (2h before other medications) and qhs. [Generic/Trade: tab 1g. Trade only: susp 1g/10ml.] ▶Not absorbed ♀B ◗? $$$

Antiulcer - Proton Pump Inhibitors

lansoprazole (*Prevacid*): Duodenal ulcer or maintenance therapy after healing of duodenal ulcer, or erosive esophagitis, GERD: 15 mg PO qd. Erosive esophagitis or gastric ulcer: 30 mg PO qd. [Trade only: cap 15,30.] ▶L ♀B ◗? $$$$

omeprazole (*Prilosec, Losec*): Duodenal ulcer or erosive esophagitis: 20 mg PO qd. Gastric ulcer: 40 mg PO qd. Hypersecretory conditions: 60 mg PO qd. [Trade only: cap 10,20,40.] ▶L ♀C ◗? $$$$

pantoprazole (*Protonix, Pantoloc*): 40 mg PO qd. [Trade only: tab 40] ▶L ♀B ◗? $$$

rabeprazole (*Aciphex*): 20 mg PO qd. [Trade only: tab 20.] ▶L ♀B ◗? $$$$

Laxatives

bisacodyl (*Correctol, Dulcolax, Feen-a-Mint*): 10-15 mg PO prn, 10 mg PR prn, 5-10 mg PR prn if 2-11 yo. [Generic/Trade: tab 5, supp 10.] ▶L ♀+ ◗? $

cascara: 325 mg PO qhs prn or 5ml of aromatic fluid extract PO qhs prn. [Generic: tab 325, liquid aromatic fluid extract.] ▶L ♀C ◗+ $

castor oil (*Purge, Fleet Flavored Castor Oil*): 15-30 ml of castor oil or 30-60 ml emulsified castor oil PO qhs, 5-15 ml/dose of castor oil PO or 7.5-30 ml emulsified castor oil PO for child. [Generic/Trade: liquid 30,60,120,480 ml, emulsified susp 45,60,90,120ml.] ▶Not absorbed ♀- ◗? $

docusate calcium (*Surfak*): 240 mg PO qd. Peds: 50-150 mg/d. [Generic/Trade: cap 240. Trade only: cap 50.] ▶L ♀+ ◗? $

docusate sodium (*Colace*): 50-400 mg/day PO divided in 1-4 doses. Peds: 10-40 mg/d if <3 yo, 20-60 mg/d if 3-6 yo, 40-150 mg/d if 6-12 yo. [Generic/Trade: cap 50,100, 240,250, tab 50,100, liquid 10 & 50 mg/5ml, syrup 16.75 & 20 mg/5ml.] ▶L ♀+ ◗? $

glycerin: one adult or infant supp PR prn. [Generic/Trade: supp infant & adult, solution (Fleet Babylax) 4 ml/applicator.] ▶Not absorbed ♀C ◗? $

lactulose (*Chronulac, Cephulac, Acilac*): Constipation: 15-30 ml PO qhs. Hepatic encephalopathy: 30-45 ml PO tid/qid, or 300 ml retention enema. [Generic/Trade: syrup 10g/15ml.] ▶Not absorbed ♀B ◗? $$

magnesium citrate: 150- 300 ml PO divided qd-bid. Children < 6 yo: 2-4 ml/kg/24h. [Generic: solution 300ml/bottle.] ▶K ♀+ ◗? $

magnesium hydroxide (*Milk of Magnesia*): Laxative: 30-60 ml regular strength liquid PO. Antacid: 5-15 ml regular strength liquid or 622-1244 mg PO qid prn. [Generic/Trade: liquid 400 & 800 (concentrated) mg/5ml, chew tab 311.] ▶K ♀+ ◗? $

methylcellulose (*Citrucel*): 1 heaping tablespoon in 8 oz. water PO qd-tid. [Trade only: Packets, multiple use canisters.] ▶Not absorbed ♀+ ◗? $

mineral oil (*Agoral, Kondremul, Fleet Mineral Oil Enema*): 15-45 ml PO. Peds: 5-20 ml/dose PO. Mineral oil enema: 120 ml PR. Peds 30-60 ml PR. [Generic/Trade: plain mineral oil, mineral oil emulsion (Agoral, Kondremul).] ▶Not absorbed ♀C ◗? $

Peri-Colace (docusate/casanthranol): 1-2 caps (100/30) PO qhs prn, 15-30 ml liquid (60/30 per 15ml) PO qhs prn. Peds: 5-15 ml PO qhs prn. [Generic/Trade: cap 100/30 mg, syrup 60/30mg per 15ml.] ▶L ♀C ◗? $

polycarbophil (*FiberCon, Fiberall, Equalactin*): Laxative: 1g PO qid prn. Diarrhea: 1g PO q30 min. Max daily dose 6g. [Generic/Trade: tab 500,625, chew tab 500,1000.] ▶Not absorbed ♀+ ◗? $

polyethylene glycol (*Miralax*): 1 heaping tsp. in 8 oz. water PO qd. [Trade only: powder for oral solution.] ▶Not absorbed ♀C ◗? $

polyethylene glycol with electrolytes (*GoLytely, CoLytely, Klean-Prep, Lyteprep*): Bowel prep: 240 ml q10 min PO or 20-30 ml/min per NG until 4L is consumed. [Generic/Trade: powder for oral solution.] ▶Not absorbed ♀C ◗? $

psyllium (*Metamucil, Fiberall, Hydrocil*): 1 tsp in liquid; 1 packet or 1-2 wafers with liquid PO qd-tid. [Generic/Trade: powder, granules, wafers.] ▶Not absorbed ♀+ ◗? $

senna (*Senokot*): 2 tabs or 1 tsp granules or 10-15 ml syrup PO or 1 supp PR qhs. Max 8 tabs, 4 tsp granules, 30 ml syrup or 2 supp per day. Take granules with full glass of water. [Generic/Trade: granules 326 mg/tsp, supp 652, syrup 218mg/5ml, tab 187,217,374,600.] ▶L ♀C ◗+ $

sodium phosphate (*Fleet enema, Fleet Phospho-Soda, Gent-L-Tip*): 1 adult or pediatric enema PR or 20-30 ml of oral soln PO prn. [Trade only: pediatric & adult enema, oral solution.] ▶Not absorbed ♀+ ◗? $

sorbitol: 30-150 ml (of 70% solution) PO or 120 ml (of 25-30% solution) PR as a single dose. [Generic: solution 70%.] ▶Not absorbed ♀+ ◗? $

Other GI Agents

alosetron (*Lotronex*): 1 mg PO bid. [Trade only: tab 1.] ▶L ♀B ◗? $$$$

balsalazide (*Colazal*): 750 mg PO TID x 8-12 weeks. [Trade: cap 750 mg .] ▶Minimal absorption ♀B ◗? ?

cisapride (*Propulsid*): 10mg PO qid, at least 15 min before meals and qhs. Available only through limited-access protocol through manufacturer. Can cause potentially fatal cardiac arrhythmias. Many drug and disease interactions. [Trade: Tab 10,20, susp 1mg/1ml.] ▶LK ♀C ◗? $$$

infliximab (*Remicade*): 5 mg/kg IV infusion. May be repeated at 2 & 6 weeks for fistualizing Crohn's disease. ▶Serum ♀C ◗? $$$$$

lactase enzyme (*Lactaid*): Swallow or chew 3 caplets (Original strength), 2 caplets (Extra strength), 1 caplet (Ultra) with first bite of dairy foods. Adjust dose based on response. [Trade only: caplets (Original, Extra strength, Ultra), chew tab (Ultra).] ▶Not absorbed ♀+ ◗+ $

Librax (clinidium + chlordiazepoxide): 1 cap PO tid-qid. [Generic/Trade: cap clinidium 2.5 mg + chlordiazepoxide 5 mg.] ▶K ♀D ◗- $

mesalamine (*Asacol, Pentasa, Rowasa, Mesasal*): Asacol: 800 mg PO tid. Pentasa: 1000 mg PO qid. Rowasa: 500 mg PR bid or 4g enema qhs [Trade only: delayed release tab 400 (Asacol), controlled release cap 250 (Pentasa), supp 500 (Rowasa), rectal susp 4g/60ml (Rowasa).] ▶Gut ♀B ◗? $$$$

neomycin (*Mycifradin*): Hepatic encephalopathy: 4-12 g/day PO divided q6-8h. Peds: 50-100 mg/kg/day PO divided q6-8h. [Generic/Trade: tab 500, solution 125mg/5ml.] ▶Not absorbed ♀D ◗? $$$

octreotide (*Sandostatin*): Variceal bleeding: Bolus 25-50 mcg IV followed by infusion 25-50 mcg/hr. AIDS diarrhea: 100-500 mcg SC tid. Other indications with varying doses. [Trade only: vials for injection 0.05,0.1,0.2,0.5,1 mg.] ▶LK ♀B ◗? $$$$$

olsalazine (*Dipentum*): Ulcerative colitis: 500 mg PO bid. [Trade only: cap 250.] ▶L ♀C ◗- $$$$

orlistat (*Xenical*): Weight loss: 120 mg PO tid with meals. [Trade only: cap 120.] ▶Gut ♀B ◗? $$$$

pancreatin (*Creon, Donnazyme, Entozyme*): 8,000-24,000 units lipase (1-2 tab/cap) PO with meals and snacks. [Tab, cap with varying amounts of pancreatin, lipase, amylase and protease.] ▶Gut ♀C ◗? $$$

pancrelipase (*Viokase, Pancrease, Cotazym, Ku-Zyme*): 4,000-33,000 units lipase (1-3 tab/cap) PO with meals and snacks. [Tab, cap, powder with varying amounts of lipase, amylase and protease.] ▶Gut ♀C ◗? $$$

sibutramine (*Meridia*): 10mg PO qd; can increase to 15mg qd after 4 weeks. [Trade only: cap 5,10,15.] ▶L ♀C ◗- $$$

sulfasalazine (*Azulfidine, Azulfidine EN-tabs, Salazopyrin, Salazopyrin EN*): 500-1000 mg PO qid. Peds: 30-60 mg/kg/day divided q4-6h. [Con/Trad: tab 500.] ▶K ♀- ◗? $$

ursodiol (*Actigall, Ursofalk, Urso*): 8-10 mg/kg/day PO divided bid/tid. [Trade only: cap 300.] ▶Bile ♀B ◗? $$$$

vasopressin (*Pitressin, ADH*): Variceal bleeding: 0.2-0.4 units/min initially (max 0.9 units/min). ▶LK ♀C ◗? $$$$$

HEMATOLOGY (See cardiology section for antiplatelet drugs and thrombolytics)

Anticoagulants - Low-Molecular-Weight Heparins & Heparinoids

ardeparin (*Normiflo*): DVT prophylaxis, knee replacement: 50 anti-Xa units/kg SC q12h starting 12-24 h postop x ≤14 days or until ambulatory. ▶LK ♀C ◗? $$$$$

dalteparin (*Fragmin*): DVT prophylaxis, abdominal surgery: 2,500 units SC 1-2 hours preop & qd postop x 5-10d. DVT prophylaxis, abdominal surgery in patients with malignancy: 5,000 units SC evening before surgery and qd postop x 5-10 days. DVT prophylaxis, hip replacement: 2,500 units SC 2 hours preop and 2,500 units SC in the evening after surgery (≥6h after first dose), then 5,000 units SC qd for up to 14 days. Unstable angina or non-Q-wave MI: 120 units/kg up to 10,000 units SC q12h with aspirin (75-165 mg/day PO) until clinically stable. ▶LK ♀B ◗? $$$$$

danaparoid (*Orgaran*): DVT prophylaxis, hip replacement: 750 anti-Xa units SC q12h starting 1-4 h preop x 7-10 days. Second dose not <2 h postop. ▶K ♀B ◗? $$$$$

enoxaparin (*Lovenox*): DVT prophylaxis for hip/knee surgery: 30 mg SC q12h starting 12-24 h postop. Alternative for hip replacement: 40 mg SC qd starting 12h preop. Abdominal surgery: 40 mg SC qd starting 2 h preop. Outpatient treatment of DVT without pulmonary embolus: 1.0 mg/kg SC q12h until PO anticoagulation established. Inpatient treatment of DVT with/without pulmonary embolus: 1 mg/kg SC q12h or 1.5 mg/kg SC q24h. Unstable angina or non-Q-wave MI: 1 mg/kg SC q12h with aspirin (100-325 mg PO qd) for ≥2 days and until clinically stable. [Trade: Prefilled syringes 30,40; graduated prefilled syringes 60,80,100; ampules 30.] ▶LK ♀B ◗? $$$$$

tinzaparin (*Innohep*): DVT with/without pulmonary embolus: 175 anti-Xa units/kg SC qd for at least 6 days and until adequate anticoagulation with warfarin. ▶K ♀B ◗? ?

Anticoagulants - Other

heparin (*Hepalean*): Load 80 units/kg IV, then mix infusion 25,000 units in 250 ml D5W (100 units/ml) and start at 18 units/kg/hour. 63 kg adult: Load 5,000 units, then run infusion at 11 ml/h. Adjust based on coags (PTT). DVT prophylaxis: 5000 units SC q8-12h. Peds: Load 50 units/kg IV, then 25 units/kg/h infusion. ▶LK ♀C but + ▶+ $$

lepirudin (*Refludan*): Thromboembolism in heparin-induced thrombocytopenia: Bolus 0.4 mg/kg up to 44 mg IV over 15-20 seconds followed by infusion of 0.15 mg/kg/hr up to 16.5 mg/h. ▶K ♀B ▶? $$$$$

warfarin (*Coumadin, Warfilone*): Start 5 mg PO qd x 2-4 days, then adjust dose to PT/INR. Higher loading doses no longer recommended. [Generic/Trade: Tabs 1,2,2.5,3,4,5,6,7.5,10.] ▶L ♀X ▶+ $

Other Hematological Agents (See endocrine section for vitamins and minerals)

aminocaproic acid (*Amicar*): 4-5 g PO/IV over 1h, then 1 g/h as needed. [Generic/Trade: Syrup 250 mg/ml. Trade: Tabs 500.] ▶K ♀D ▶? $$

cilostazol (*Pletal*): Claudication: 100 mg PO bid on empty stomach. 50 mg PO bid with ketoconazole, itraconazole, erythromycin, diltiazem, omeprazole. Avoid grapefruit juice. [Trade: Tabs 50, 100.] ▶L ♀C ▶? $$$

desmopressin (*DDAVP, Stimate*): Hemophilia A, von Willebrand's disease: 0.3 mcg/ kg IV over 15-30 min, or 150-300 mcg intranasally. [Trade: Nasal spray 150 mcg/0.1 ml.] ▶LK ♀B ▶? $$$$$

erythropoietin (*Epogen, Procrit, epoetin alfa, Eprex*): Anemia: 1 dose IV/SC 3 times/ week. Initial dose if renal failure = 50-100 units/kg, AZT = 100 units/kg, or chemo = 150 units/kg. ▶L ♀C ▶? $$$$$

factor VIII, IX: specialized dosing. ▶L ♀C ▶? $$$$$

filgrastim (*G-CSF, Neupogen*): Neutropenia: 5 mcg/kg SC/IV qd. [Trade: Single-dose vials 300 mcg/1 ml, 480 mcg/1.6 ml.] ▶L ♀C ▶? $$$$$

oprelvekin (*Neumega*): Thrombocytopenia: 50 mcg/kg (adults) or 75-100 mcg/kg (peds) SC qd. ▶K ♀C ▶? $$$$$

pentoxifylline (*Trental*): 400 mg PO tid with meals. [Gen/Trade: Tabs 400.] ▶L ♀C ▶? $$

protamine: Reversal of heparin: 1 mg antagonizes ~100 units heparin. Beware of allergy/anaphylaxis. ▶Plasma ♀C ▶? $

sargramostim (*GM-CSF, Leukine*): Specialized marrow transplant dose.▶L♀C▶? $$$$$

IMMUNOLOGY

Immunizations

BCG vaccine (*Tice BCG*): 0.2-0.3 ml multidose puncture disc. ▶? ♀C ▶? $$$$

cholera vaccine (*Cholera vaccine, USP*): 0.2 ml ID x 2 doses. ▶? ♀C ▶? $

Comvax (haemophilus b + hepatitis B vaccine): 0.5 ml IM. ▶L ♀C ▶? $$$

diphtheria, tetanus, and acellular pertussis vaccine (*DTaP, Tripedia, Acel-Imune, Infanrix, Certiva*): 0.5 ml IM. ▶L ♀C ▶- $

diphtheria-tetanus toxoid (*Td,DT*): 0.5 ml IM. [injection DT (pediatric: 6 weeks- 6 yo). Td (adult and children: ≥7 years).] ▶L ♀C ▶? $

haemophilus b vaccine (*ActHIB, HibTITER, OmniHIB, PedvaxHIB, ProHIBit*): 0.5 ml IM. ▶L ♀C ▶? $

hepatitis A vaccine (*Havrix, Vaqta*): Adult formulation 1 ml IM, repeat in 6-12 months. Peds doses vary by brand. ▶L ♀C ▶? $$$

hepatitis B vaccine (*Engerix-B, Recombivax HB*): Adults: 1 ml IM, repeat in 1 and 6 months. Separate pediatric formulations and dosing. ▶L ♀C ▶? $$$

influenza vaccine (*Fluzone, Fluvirin, FluShield, Fluogen, Fluviral, Vaxigrip*): 0.5 ml IM. ▶L ♀C ◗+ $

Japanese encephalitis vaccine (*JE-Vax*): 1.0 ml SC x 3 doses on days 0, 7, and 30. ▶? ♀C ◗? $$$$$

lymo disease vaccine (*LYMErix*): 30 mcg IM, repeat in 1 & 12 months. ▶L ♀C ◗? $$$

measles, mumps and rubella vaccine (*M-M-R II*): 0.5 ml (1 vial) SC. ▶L ♀C ◗? $$

meningococcal polysaccharide vaccine (*Menomune-A/C/Y/W 135*): 0.5 ml SC ▶? ♀C ◗? $$$

plague vaccine (*Plague vaccine*): Age 18-61 yo: 1 ml IM x 1 dose, then 0.2 ml IM 1-3 mon after the 1st injection, then 0.2 ml IM 5-6 mon after 2nd injection. ▶? ♀C ◗+ $

pneumococcal 7-valent conjugate vaccine (*Prevnar*): 0.5 ml IM x 3 doses 6-8 weeks apart starting at 2-6 mon of age, followed by a 4th dose at 12-15 mon. ▶L ♀C ◗? $$$

pneumococcal vaccine (*Pneumovax, Pnu-Imune, Pneumo 23*): 0.5 ml IM/SC.▶L♀C◗? $

poliovirus vaccine (*Sabin: Orimune; inactivated: IPOL*): An all-IPV schedule is recommended. Inactivated (IPOL): 0.5 ml SC. ▶L ♀C ◗? $$

rabies vaccine (*RabAvert, Imovax*): 1 ml IM on days 0, 3, 7, 14, 28. ▶L ♀C ◗? $$$$$

tetanus toxoid: 0.5 ml IM/SC. ▶L ♀C ◗? $

TriHibit (haemophilus b + DTaP): 4th dose only, 15-18 mos; 0.5 ml IM. ▶L ♀C ◗- $$

typhoid vaccine (*Vivotif Berna, Typhim Vi, Typhoid Vaccine, USP*): 0.5 ml IM x 1 dose (Typhim Vi); 0.5 ml SC x 2 doses (Typhoid Vaccine, USP); 1 cap qod x 4 doses. May revaccinate q2-5 yrs in high risk patients. [Trade only: Caps] ▶? ♀C ◗? $$

varicella vaccine (*Varivax*): Children 1 to 12 yo: 0.5 ml SC x 1 dose. Age ≥13: 0.5 ml SC, repeat 4-8 weeks later. ▶L ♀C ◗? $$$

yellow fever vaccine (*YF-Vax*): 0.5 ml SC ▶? ♀C ◗+ $$$

<table>
<tr><th colspan="10">CHILDHOOD IMMUNIZATION SCHEDULE* Months</th><th colspan="3">Years</th></tr>
<tr><th>Age</th><th>Birth</th><th>1</th><th>2</th><th>4</th><th>6</th><th>12</th><th>15</th><th>18</th><th>24</th><th>4-6</th><th>11-12</th><th>14-16</th></tr>
<tr><td rowspan="2">Hepatitis B</td><td colspan="3">HB-1</td><td colspan="9"></td></tr>
<tr><td></td><td colspan="3">HB-2</td><td colspan="4">HB-3</td><td colspan="4"></td></tr>
<tr><td>DPT†</td><td></td><td></td><td>DTP</td><td>DTP</td><td>DTP</td><td></td><td colspan="2">DTP</td><td></td><td>DTP</td><td colspan="2">Td</td></tr>
<tr><td>H influenza b</td><td></td><td></td><td>Hib</td><td>Hib</td><td>Hib</td><td colspan="2">Hib</td><td></td><td></td><td></td><td></td><td></td></tr>
<tr><td>Pneumococci</td><td></td><td></td><td>Pne</td><td>Pne</td><td>Pne</td><td colspan="2">Pne</td><td></td><td></td><td></td><td></td><td></td></tr>
<tr><td>Polio§</td><td></td><td></td><td>IPV</td><td>IPV</td><td colspan="4">IPV</td><td></td><td>IPV</td><td></td><td></td></tr>
<tr><td>MMR</td><td></td><td></td><td></td><td></td><td></td><td colspan="2">MMR</td><td></td><td></td><td>MMR</td><td></td><td></td></tr>
<tr><td>Varicella</td><td></td><td></td><td></td><td></td><td></td><td colspan="3">Varicella</td><td></td><td></td><td></td><td></td></tr>
<tr><td>Hepatitis A¶</td><td></td><td></td><td></td><td></td><td></td><td></td><td></td><td></td><td colspan="3">HA (some areas)</td><td></td></tr>
</table>

*2000 schedule from the CDC, ACIP, AAP, & AAFP, amended to include new pneumococcal vaccine; see www.aap.org/family/parents/immunize.htm for updates & expanded discussion, including catch-up doses. †Acellular form preferred for all DTP doses. §Inactivated form (IPV) preferred for all doses. ¶Recommended for selected high-risk areas, consult local public health authorities.

Immunoglobulins

hepatitis B immune globulin (*H-BIG, BayHep B, NABI-HB*): 0.06 ml/kg IM within 24 hours of needlestick, ocular, or mucosal exposure, repeat in 1 month. ▶L ♀C ◗? $$$

immune globulin (*Gamimune, Polygam, Sandoglobulin, Gammagard, Gammar, Venoglobulin, Baygam*): IV dosage varies by indication. IM form (Baygam): Hepatitis A protection (up to 3 months): 0.02 ml/kg IM. Measles (within 6 days post-exposure): 0.2-0.25 ml/kg IM. ▶L ♀C ◗? $$$$$

rabies immune globulin, human (*Imogam, BayRab*): 20 units/kg, as much as possible infiltrated around bite, the rest IM. ▶L ♀C ▶? $$$$$

RHO immune globulin (*RhoGAM, BayRho-D, WinRho SDF*): 1 vial IM within 72h if mother Rh-. ▶L ♀C ▶? $$$$

RSV immune globulin (*RespiGam*): IV infusion for peds RSV. ▶Plasma ♀C ▶? $$$$$

tetanus immune globulin (*BayTet*): Prophylaxis: 250 units IM. ▶L ♀C ▶? $$$$

varicella-zoster immune globulin (*VZIG*): Specialized dosing. ▶L ♀C ▶? $$$$$

Immunosuppression

basiliximab (*Simulect*): Specialized transplantation dosing. ▶Plasma ♀B ▶? $$$$$

cyclosporine (*Sandimmune, Neoral, SangCYA*): Specialized transplant dosing. [Trade: Caps (Sand.) 25,100 mg. microemulsion Caps (Neoral) 25, 100 mg. Sol'n (Sand.) 100 mg/ml. microemulsion sol'n (Neoral, SangCYA) 100 mg/ml.] ▶L ♀C ▶- $$$$$

daclizumab (*Zenapax*): Specialized transplant dosing: 1 mg/kg IV. ▶L ♀C ▶? $$$$$

mycophenolate mofetil (*Cellcept*): Specialized transplant dosing. [Trade only: Caps 250 mg. Tabs 500 mg.] ▶? ♀C ▶? $$$$$

sirolimus (*Rapamune*): Specialized transplant dosing. [Trade: oral solution 1 mg/ml.] ▶L ♀C ▶- $$$$$

tacrolimus (*Prograf, FK 506*): Specialized transplant dosing. [Trade only: Caps 1,5 mg.] ▶L ♀C ▶- $$$$$

Other

tuberculin PPD (*Aplisol, Tubersol, Mantoux, PPD*): 5 TU intradermally, read 48-72h later. ▶L ♀C ▶+ $

NEUROLOGY

Alzheimer's Dementia

NOTE: Used for mild to moderate (Folstein MMSE 10-26) Alzheimer's dementia.

donepezil (*Aricept*): Start 5 mg PO hs. May increase to 10 mg PO hs in 4-6 wks. [Trade: Tabs 5, 10 mg.] ▶LK ♀C ▶? $$$$

rivastigmine (*Exelon*): Start 1.5 mg PO bid, increase to 3 mg bid after 2 weeks. Max 12 mg/day. [Trade: Caps 1.5, 3, 4.5, 6 mg. Oral solution 2 mg/ml.] ▶L ♀B ▶? $$$$

tacrine (*Cognex*): 10 mg PO qid for 4 weeks (monitor LFT's q2 weeks), then increase to 20 mg qid. Titrate to higher doses q4 weeks based on tolerability. Hepatotoxicity. [Trade: Caps 10, 20, 30, 40 mg.] ▶L ♀C ▶? $$$$

Anticonvulsants

carbamazepine (*Tegretol, Tegretol XR, Carbatrol, Epitol, Mazepine*): 200-400 mg PO bid-qid. Extended release: 200 mg PO bid. Aplastic anemia. [Generic/Trade: Tabs 200 mg. chewable Tabs 100 mg. Trade only: extended release Tabs 100, 200, 300, 400 mg. susp 100 mg/ 5 ml.] ▶LK ♀D ▶+ $

clonazepam (*Klonopin, Rivotril, Clonapam*): Start 0.5 mg PO tid, max 20 mg/d. [Generic/Trade: Tabs 0.5, 1, 2 mg.] ▶LK ♀D ▶? ©IV $$$

diazepam (*Valium, Diastat, Vivol, E Pam*): Active seizing: 0.2-0.4 mg/kg up to 5-30 mg IV, or 0.2-0.5 mg/kg rectal gel PR. [Generic/Trade: Tabs 2, 5, 10 mg. solution 5 mg/ 5 ml. Trade only: concentrated solution (Intensol) 5 mg/ml. rectal gel (Diastat) 2.5, 5, 10, 15, 20 mg.] ▶K ♀D ▶- ©IV $

ethosuximide (*Zarontin*): 250 mg PO qd or divided bid if 3-6 yo, 500 mg PO qd or divided bid if >6 yo. [Trade only: Caps 250 mg. Generic/Trade: syrup 250 mg/ 5ml.] ▶LK ♀C ▶+ $$$$

felbamate (*Felbatol*): Start 400 mg PO tid, max 3600 mg/day. Peds: Start 15 mg/kg/ day PO, max 45 mg/kg/day. Aplastic anemia, hepatotoxicity. [Trade: Tabs 400, 600 mg. susp 600 mg/ 5 ml.] ▶KL ♀C ▶- $$$$

fosphenytoin (*Cerebyx*): Load 15-20 mg "phenytoin equivalents" per kg either IM, or IV no faster than 100-150 mg/min. ▶L ♀D ▶+ $$$$$

gabapentin (*Neurontin*): Start 300 mg PO hs, and increase over a few days to 300-600 mg PO tid, maximum 3600 mg/day. [Trade: Caps 100, 300, 400 mg. Tabs 600, 800 mg. solution 50 mg/ml.] ▶K ♀C ▶? $$$$

lamotrigine (*Lamictal, Lamictal CD*): Start 50 mg PO qd x 2 wks, then 50 mg bid x 2 wks, then maintenance 150-250 mg PO bid. Life-threatening rashes in 1:1000 adults & 1:50 children. See product labeling for dose adjustment when used with valproic acid. [Trade: Tabs 25, 100, 150, 200 mg. chewable Tabs 5, 25 mg.] ▶LK ♀C ▶- $$$$

levetiracetam (*Keppra*): Start 500 mg PO bid, titrate to maximum dose of 3000 mg/ day. [Trade: Tabs 250, 500, 750 mg.] ▶LK ♀C ▶? $$$$$

lorazepam (*Ativan*): active seizure: 0.05-0.1 mg/kg IV over 2-5 min. ▶LK ♀D ▶- ©IV $$$

oxcarbazepine (*Trileptal*): Start 300 mg PO bid, titrate to 1200 mg/ day (adjunctive) or 1200- 2400 mg/ day (monotherapy). Peds age 4-16 yo: start 8- 10 mg/kg/day divided bid. [Trade: Tabs 150, 300, 600 mg.] ▶L ♀C ▶- $$$$

phenobarbital (*Luminal*): Load 200- 600 mg IV at rate ≤60 mg/min up to total dose of 20 mg/kg. Maintenance 100-300 mg/day PO, peds 3-5 mg/kg/day PO divided bid/tid. Multiple drug interactions. [Generic/Trade: Tabs 15, 16, 30, 32, 60, 65, 100 mg. elixir 20 mg/5ml.] ▶L ♀D ▶- ©IV $

phenytoin (*Dilantin, Diphen, Tremytoine*): Load 10-20 mg/kg (1000 mg in typical adult) IV no faster than 50 mg/min. Oral load: 400 mg PO initially, then 300 mg in 2h & 4h. Maintenance: 5 mg/kg or 300 mg PO qd or divided tid. QD dosing only with Dilantin brand Caps. [Generic/Trade: Caps 100 mg. susp 125 mg/ 5 ml. ext release Caps 100 mg. Trade only: extended release Caps 30 mg. chewable Tabs 50 mg.] ▶L ♀D ▶+ $

primidone (*Mysoline, Sertan*): Start 100-125 mg PO hs, increase over 10d to 250 mg tid/ qid. Metabolized to phenobarbital. [Trade only: Tabs 50 mg. susp 250 mg/ 5 ml. Generic/Trade: Tabs 250 mg.] ▶LK ♀D ▶- $

tiagabine (*Gabitril*): Start 4 mg PO qd, and gradually increase prn to max 32 mg/ day (children) or 56 mg/d (adults) divided bid-qid. [Trade: Tabs 2, 4, 12, 16, 20 mg.] ▶LK ♀C ▶- $$$$

topiramate (*Topamax*): Start 50 mg PO hs, then increase by 50 mg/d (divided doses) once weekly to usual effective dose of 200 mg bid. [Trade only: Tabs 25, 100, 200 mg. sprinkle Caps 15, 25 mg.] ▶K ♀C ▶? $$$$$

valproic acid (*Depakene, Depakote, Depacon, Deproic, Epiject, Epival*): Seizures: 10-15 mg/kg/d PO/IV, titrate to max 60 mg/kg/d. Parenteral (Depacon): ≤20 mg/min IV. Hepatotoxicity, drug interactions, reduce dose in elderly. [Trade only: Tabs, delayed release (Depakote) 125,250,500 mg. Caps, sprinkle (Depakote) 125 mg. Generic/ Trade: syrup (Depakene) 250 mg/ 5 ml. Caps (Depakene) 250 mg.] ▶L ♀D ▶+ $$$$

zonisamide (*Zonegran*): Start 100 mg PO qd, titrate q2 weeks up to 300-400 mg/ day qd or divided bid. Max 600 mg/ day. Contraindicated in patients allergic to sulfonamides. [Trade: Caps 100 mg.] ▶LK ♀C ▶- $$$$

Migraine Therapy - 5-HT1 Receptor Agonists

NOTE: Avoid with coronary artery disease, uncontrolled HTN, & ergot drugs.

naratriptan (*Amerge*): 1-2.5 mg PO, may repeat in 4h for maximum daily dose of 5 mg. [Trade: Tabs 1, 2.5 mg.] ▶KL ♀C ▶? $$

rizatriptan (*Maxalt, Maxalt MLT*): 5-10 mg PO, may repeat in 2h, max dose 30 mg/24h. MLT form dissolves on tongue without liquids. [Trade: Tabs 5, 10 mg. orally disintegrating Tabs (MLT) 5, 10 mg.] ▶LK ♀C ▶? $$

sumatriptan (*Imitrex*): 6 mg SC, may repeat after 1h, max 12 mg/day. 25 mg PO, may repeat q2h with 25-100 mg doses to max of 200-300 mg/day. 5-20 mg intranasal spray q2h to max 40 mg/day. [Trade: Tabs 25, 50 mg. nasal spray 5, 20 mg/ spray. injection 6 mg/0.5 ml.] ▶K ♀C ▶? $$

zolmitriptan (*Zomig*): 1.25-2.5 mg PO q2h, max 10 mg/24 hours. [Trade: Tabs 2.5, 5 mg.] ▶L ♀C ▶? $$

Migraine Therapy - Other

Cafergot, Ercaf, Wigraine (ergotamine/caffeine): 2 tabs (1/100 mg each) PO at onset, then 1 q30 min up to 6 tabs/attack. Supp (2/100mg): up to 2 per attack. [Trade: Tabs 1/100 mg. Supp 2/100.] ▶L ♀X ▶- $

dihydroergotamine (*DHE 45, Migranal*): 1 mg IV/IM/SC, repeat in 1h prn; max 2 mg (IV) or 3 mg (IM/SC) per day. Nasal (Migranal): 1 spray in each nostril, repeat 15 mins later. Max 6 sprays/24h and 8 sprays/wk. [Trade: nasal 0.5 mg/ spray.] ▶L ♀X ▶- $$

Duradrin, Midrin (isometheptene /dichloralphenazone/acetaminophen): 2 tabs PO followed by 1 per hour until relief, up to 5 per 12-hour period. [Trade: Caps 65 mg isometheptene/ 100 mg dichloralphenazone/ 325 mg acetaminophen] ▶L ♀? ▶? $

Excedrin Migraine (acetaminophen/aspirin/caffeine): 2 Tabs PO q6h, max 8 tabs/d. [OTC/Generic/Trade: Tabs 250/250/65 mg.] ▶LK ♀D ▶? $

valproic acid (*Depakene, Depakote, Deproic, Epiject, Epival*): Migraine prophylaxis: 250 mg PO bid. Hepatotoxicity, drug interactions, reduce dose in elderly. [Trade: Tabs, delayed release (Depakote) 125,250,500. Caps, sprinkle (Depakote) 125 mg. Generic/Trade: syrup (Depakene) 250 mg/ 5 ml. Caps (Depakene) 250 mg.] ▶L ♀D ▶+ $$

Parkinsonian Agents - Anticholinergics

benztropine mesylate (*Cogentin, Bensylate*): 0.5-2 mg IM/PO/IV qd/bid. [Generic/ Trade: Tabs 0.5, 1, 2 mg.] ▶LK ♀C ▶? $

biperiden (*Akineton*): 2 mg PO tid/qid or 2 mg IV/IM q30 min prn. [Trade: Tabs 2 mg] ▶LK ♀C ▶? $$

trihexyphenidyl (*Artane, Aparkane*): Start 1 mg/day PO, then increase slowly to 6-10 mg/day, divided tid. Max 15 mg/day. [Generic/Trade: Tabs 2, 5 mg. elixir 2 mg/ 5ml.] ▶LK ♀C ▶? $

Parkinsonian Agents - COMT Inhibitors

entacapone (*Comtan*): Start 200 mg PO as adjunct to levodopa/carbidopa, max 8 times/day (1600 mg). [Trade: Tabs 200 mg.] ▶L ♀C ▶? $$$$

tolcapone (*Tasmar*): Start 100 mg PO tid, only as an adjunct to levodopa/carbidopa. Max 600 mg/day. Hepatotoxicity, monitor LFTs. [Trade: Tabs 100, 200 mg.] ▶LK ♀C ▶? $$$$

Parkinsonian Agents - Dopaminergic Agents

amantadine (*Symmetrel, Endantadine*): 100 mg PO bid. [Trade only: Tabs 100 mg. Generic: Caps 100 mg. Generic/Trade: syrup 50 mg/ 5ml.] ▶K ♀C ◗- $

Atamet (carbidopa/levodopa): Start 1 tab PO tid, then increase q1-4 days as needed to max 200 mg/day carbidopa. [Generic/Trade: Tabs 25/100, 25/250.] ▶L ♀C ◗- $$$

bromocriptine (*Parlodel*): Start 1.25 mg PO bid, usual effective dose 10-40 mg/day, max 100 mg/day. [Generic/Trade: Tabs 2.5 mg. Caps 5 mg.] ▶L ♀B ◗ $$$$

levodopa (*Laradopa*): Start 250-500 mg PO bid, max 8g/day. [Trade: Tabs 100, 250, 500 mg.] ▶L ♀- ◗- $$

pergolide (*Permax*): Start 0.05 mg PO qd, then gradually increase to 1 mg PO tid. Maximum 5 mg/day. [Trade: Tabs 0.05, 0.25, 1 mg.] ▶K ♀B ◗? $$$$$

pramipexole (*Mirapex*): Start 0.125 mg PO tid, then gradually increase to 0.5-1.5 mg PO tid. [Trade: Tabs 0.125, 0.25, 1, 1.5 mg.] ▶K ♀C ◗? $$$$

ropinirole (*Requip*): Start 0.25 mg PO tid, then gradually increase to 1 mg PO tid. Maximum 24 mg/day. [Trade: Tabs 0.25, 0.5, 1, 2, 4, 5 mg.] ▶L ♀C ◗? $$$

selegiline (*Eldepryl, Atapryl, Carbex, Selpak*): 5 mg PO q am and q noon. [Generic/Trade: Caps 5 mg. Tabs 5 mg.] ▶LK ♀C ◗? $$$

Sinemet (carbidopa/levodopa): Start 1 tab PO tid, then increase q1-4 days prn to max 200 mg/d carbidopa. Sust'd release: Start 1 tab PO bid, increase prn. [Generic/Trade: Tabs 10/100, 25/100, 25/250. Tabs, sust'd release 25/100, 50/200.] ▶L ♀C ◗- $$$

Other Neurology Agents

Aggrenox (aspirin/dipyridamole): One capsule PO bid [Trade: Caps 25 mg aspirin/ 200 mg extended-release dipyridamole.] ▶LK ♀D ◗? $$$

alteplase (*t-PA, Activase*): Thrombolysis for acute CVA with symptoms ≤3h: 0.9 mg/ kg up to 90 mg, 10% of total dose IV bolus and remainder IV over 60 min. Multiple exclusion criteria. ▶L ♀C ◗? $$$$$

dexamethasone (*Decadron, Dexasone, Hexadrol*): Cerebral edema: Load 10- 20 mg IV/IM, then 4 mg IV/IM q6h or 1-3 mg PO tid. Bacterial meningitis: 0.15 mg/kg IV/IM q6h. [Generic/Trade: Tabs 0.25, 0.5, 0.75, 1.0, 1.5, 2, 4, 6 mg. elixir/ solution 0.5 mg/5ml. Trade only: solution concentrate 0.5 mg/ 0.5 ml] ▶L ♀C ◗- $$$

edrophonium (*Tensilon, Enlon, Reversol*): Evaluation for myasthenia gravis: 2 mg test IV, then 8 mg more after 45 sec while monitored. Duration 5-10 min. ▶Plasma ♀C ◗? $

glatiramer (*Copaxone*): Multiple sclerosis: 20 mg SC qd. [Trade: injection 20 mg single dose vial.] ▶Serum ♀B ◗? $$$$$

interferon beta-1A (*Avonex, Rebif*): Multiple sclerosis: 30 mcg (6 million units) IM q wk. [Trade: injection 33 mcg (6.6 million units) single dose vial.] ▶L ♀C ◗? $$$$$

interferon beta-1B (*Betaseron*): Multiple sclerosis: 0.25 mg (8 million units) SC qod. [Trade: injection 0.3 mg (9.6 million units) single dose vial.] ▶L ♀C ◗? $$$$$

mannitol (*Osmitrol, Resectisol*): Intracranial HTN: 0.25-2 g/kg IV over 30-60 min. ▶K ♀C ◗? $$$

meclizine (*Antivert, Bonine, Medivert, Meclicot, Meni-D, Bonamine*): Vertigo: 25 mg PO q6h prn. [Rx/OTC/Generic/Trade: Tabs 12.5, 25 mg. chewable Tabs 25 mg. Rx/ Trade only: Tabs 30, 50 mg. Caps 25 mg.] ▶L ♀B ◗? $

methylprednisolone (*Solu-Medrol, Medrol, Depo-Medrol*): Spinal cord injury: 30 mg/kg IV over 15 min, followed in 45 min by 5.4 mg/kg/h IV infusion x 23-47h. ▶L ♀C ◗- $$$$$

neostigmine (*Prostigmin*): 0.5 mg IM/SC. 15-375 mg/d PO divided. [Trade: Tabs 15 mg.] ▶L ♀C ▶? $$$

nimodipine (*Nimotop*): Subarachnoid hemorrhage (Hunt/Hess grades I-III only): 60 mg PO q4h for 21 days. [Trade: Caps 30 mg.] ▶L ♀C ▶- $$$$$

pyridostigmine (*Mestinon, Regonal*): Myasthenia gravis: 60-200 mg PO tid or 180 mg (ext release) PO qd/bid. [Trade: Tabs 60 mg. extended release Tabs 180 mg. syrup 60 mg/ 5 ml.] ▶L ♀C ▶+ $$$

riluzole (*Rilutek*): ALS: 50 mg PO q12h. [Trade: Tabs 50 mg.] ▶LK ♀C ▶- $$$$$

OB/GYN

Estrogens (see also Vaginal Preparations, Hormone Replacement Combos)

NOTE: Unopposed estrogens ↑ endometrial cancer risk in postmenopausal women.

esterified estrogens (*Menest, Estratab*): HRT: 0.3 to 1.25mg PO qd. [Trade: Tabs 0.3, 0.625, 1.25, 2.5mg.] ▶L ♀X ▶- $

estradiol (*Estrace, Estradiol*): HRT: 1-2mg PO qd for 3 wks of month or continuous with daily progestin. [Generic/Trade: Tabs, micronized 0.5,1,2mg, scored.] ▶L ♀X ▶- $

estradiol cypionate (*depGynogen, Depo-Estradiol Cypionate, DepoGen*): HRT: 1-5mg IM q3 weeks, cyclically for 3 weeks on, 1 week off. ▶L ♀X ▶- $

estradiol transdermal system (*Alora, Climara, Esclim, Estraderm, FemPatch, Vivelle, Vivelle Dot*): HRT: change patch once per week (Climara, FemPatch) or twice per week (Esclim, Estraderm, Vivelle, Vivelle Dot, Alora) for first 3 weeks of month. [Trade: Transdermal patches doses in mg/day: Climara, FemPatch (q week) 0.025, Esclim (twice/week) 0.025, 0.0375, 0.05, 0.075, 0.1; Vivelle, Vivelle Dot (twice/week) 0.0375, 0.05, 0.075, 0.1; Climara (q week) & Estraderm (twice/week) 0.05, 0.075 (Climara only), & 0.1; Alora (twice/week) 0.05, 0.075, 0.1.] ▶L ♀X ▶- $$

estradiol valerate (*Delestrogen, Gynogen L.A. 20, Valergen 20, Estra-L 40, Valergen 40*): HRT: 10-20mg IM q4 weeks. ▶L ♀X ▶- $

estrogens, conjugated (*Premarin, C.E.S., Congest*): Abnormal uterine bleeding: 25mg IV/IM q6-12h until bleeding stops. HRT: 0.3 to 1.25mg PO qd for 3 weeks of month or continuous with daily progestin. [Trade: Tabs 0.3,0.625,0.9,1.25,2.5 mg.] ▶L ♀X ▶- $

estrogens, synthetic conjugated (*Cenestin*): HRT: 0.625 to 1.25mg PO qd for 3 wks of month or continuous with daily progestin. [Trade: tabs 0.625,0.9,1.25mg.] ▶L ♀X ▶- $

estrone (*Kestrone 5, Primestrin, EstraGyn 5*): HRT 0.1-1mg IM q week, up to 2mg weekly. ▶L ♀X ▶- $

estropipate (*Ogen, Ortho-Est*): HRT: 0.625 to 5mg PO qd cyclically for 3 weeks of month or continuous with daily progestin. [Generic/Trade: Tabs 0.625, 1.25, 2.5, 5mg.] ▶L ♀X ▶- $

ethinyl estradiol (*Estinyl*): HRT: 0.02–0.05mg PO qd, cyclically or continuous with daily progestin. [Trade: Tabs 0.02, 0.05, 0.5mg.] ▶L ♀X ▶- $

GnRH Agonists

ganirelix acetate (*Antagon*): Infertility: 250mcg SC qd during the early to mid follicular phase. ▶Plasma ♀X ▶? $$$$

goserelin (*Zoladex*): Endometriosis: 3.6mg implant SC q28 days or 10.8mg implant q12 weeks X 6 mo. ▶LK ♀X ▶- $$$$$

leuprolide (*Lupron*): Endometriosis or fibroid-associated anemia: 3.75mg IM q month or 11.2mg IM q3 months, for total therapy of 6 months(endometriosis) or 3 months(fibroids). Concurrent iron for fibroid-associated anemia. ▶L ♀X ▶- $$$$$

ORAL CONTRACEPTIVES ▶L, ♀X, ◗-	Estrogen (mcg)	Progestin (mg)
Monophasic		
Genora 1/50, Nelova 1/50M, Norinyl 1+50, Ortho-Novum 1/50, Necon 1/50	50 mestranol	1 norethindrone
Ovcon-50	50 ethinyl estradiol	
Demulen 1/50, Zovia 1/50E		1 ethynodiol
Ovral, Ogestrel		0.5 norgestrel
Genora 1/35, Nelova 1/35E, Norinyl 1+35, Ortho-Novum 1/35, Necon 1/35	35 ethinyl estradiol	1 norethindrone
Brevicon, Modicon, Nelova 0.5/35E, Necon 0.5/35		0.5 norethindrone
Ovcon-35		0.4 norethindrone
Ortho-Cyclen		0.25 norgestimate
Demulen 1/35, Zovia 1/35E		1 ethynodiol
Loestrin 21 1.5/30, Loestrin Fe 1.5/30	30 ethinyl estradiol	1.5 norethindrone
Lo/Ovral, Low-Ogestrel		0.3 norgestrel
Desogen, Ortho-Cept		0.15 desogestrel
Levlen, Levora, Nordette		0.15 levonorgestrel
Loestrin 21 1/20, Loestrin Fe 1/20	20 eth estr	1 norethindrone
Alesse, Levlite		0.1 levonorgestrel
Progestin-only		
Micronor, Nor-Q.D.	none	0.35 norethindrone
Ovrette	none	0.075 norgestrel
Triphasic (estrogen & progestin contents vary)		
Tri-Norinyl, Ortho-Novum 7/7/7	ethinyl estradiol	norethindrone
Tri-Levlen, Triphasil, Trivora-28		levonorgestrel
Ortho Tri-Cyclen		norgestimate
Other		
Estrostep 28 (with Fe)	20/30/35ee	1 norethindrone

nafarelin (*Synarel*): Endometriosis: 200-400mcg intranasal bid X 6 mon. [Trade: Nasal sol'n 2mg/ml in 10ml bottle (200 mcg per spray) ~56 sprays/bottle.] ▶L ♀X ◗- $$$$$

Hormone Replacement Combinations (See also vaginal preps & estrogens)

Activella (estradiol/norethindrone): 1 tab PO qd. [Trade: Tablet 1mg/0.5mg estradiol/ norethindrone acetate in calendar dial pack dispenser.] ▶L ♀X ◗- $

CombiPatch (estradiol/norethindrone): HRT: 1 patch twice weekly. [Trade: Transdermal patch in mg/day 0.05/0.14, 0.05/0.25, 8 patches/box.] ▶L ♀X ◗- $$

Estratest (esterified estrogens/methyltestosterone): 1 tab PO qd. [Trade: Tabs 1.25mg/ 2.5mg esterified estrogens/methyltestosterone.] ▶L ♀X ◗- $$

Estratest H.S. (esterified estrogens/methyltestosterone): 1 tab PO qd. [Trade: Tabs 0.625 mg/1.25mg esterified estrogens/methyltestosterone.] ▶L ♀X ◗- $$

FemHRT 1/5 (ethinyl estradiol/norethindrone): 1 tab PO qd. [Trade: Tabs 5mcg ethinyl estradiol/1mg norethindrone, 28/blister card and 90/bottle.] ▶L ♀X ◗- $

Menogen (esterified estrogens/methyltestosterone): 1 tab PO qd. [Trade:Tabs 1.25 mg/2.5mg esterified estrogens/methyltestosterone.] ▶L ♀X ◗- $

Menogen H.S. (esterified estrogens/methyltestosterone): 1 tab PO qd. [Trade: Tabs 0.625mg/1.25mg esterified estrogens/methyltestosterone.] ▶L ♀X ◗- $

DRUGS GENERALLY ACCEPTED AS SAFE IN PREGNANCY (selected)

Analgesics: acetaminophen, hydrocodone/acetaminophen, codeine*, meperidine*, methadone*. Antimicrobials: penicillins, cephalosporins, erythromycins (not estolate), azithromycin, nystatin, clotrimazole, metronidazole**, nitrofurantoin***, *Nix*. CV: labetalol, methyldopa, hydralazine. Derm: erythromycin, clindamycin, benzoyl peroxide. Endo: insulin, liothyronine, levothyroxine. ENT: chlorpheniramine, diphenhydramine*, dimenhydrinate, dextromethorphan, guaifenesin, nasal steroids, nasal cromolyn. GI: trimethobenzamide, antacids*, simethicone, cimetidine, famotidine, ranitidine, psyllium, metoclopramide, bisacodyl, docusate, doxylamine, meclizine. Psych: fluoxetine, desipramine, doxepin. Pulmonary: short-acting inhaled beta-2 agonists, cromolyn, nedocromil, beclomethasone, budesonide, theophylline, prednisone**. Other: heparin.
**Except if used long-term or in high does at term **Except 1st trimester*
****Contraindicated at term and during labor and delivery.*

Ortho-Prefest (estradiol/norgestimate): 1 tab PO qd. [Trade: Tabs in blister packs 1mg estradiol (15 pink) & 1mg estadiol/0.09mg norgestimate (15 white).] ▶L ♀X ▶- $

Premphase (conjugated estrogens/medroxyprogesterone): 1 tab PO qd. [Trade: Tabs in EZ-Dial dispensers 0.625mg conjugated estrogens (14) & 0.625mg/5mg conjugated estrogens/medroxyprogesterone (14).] ▶L ♀X ▶- $

Prempro (conjugated estrogens/medroxyprogesterone): 1 tab PO qd. [Trade: Tabs in EZ-Dial dispensers 0.625mg/5mg or 0.625mg/2.5mg conjugated estrogens/ medroxyprogesterone.] ▶L ♀X ▶- $

Labor Induction / Cervical Ripening

dinoprostone (*PGE2, Prepidil, Cervidil*): One syringe of gel placed directly into the cervical os for cervical ripening or one insert in the posterior fornix of the vagina. [Trade: Gel (Prepidil) 0.5mg/syringe; vag insert (Cervidil) 10mg.] ▶Lung ♀C ▶? $$$$

misoprostol (*PGE1, Cytotec*): 25-100mcg intravaginally q3-4h to max 500mcg/24h. [Trade: Oral Tabs 100 & 200mcg.] ▶LK ♀X ▶- $

oxytocin (*Pitocin*): 10 units in 1000ml NS (10 milliunits/ml), start at 6-12ml/h (1-2 milliunits/min). ▶LK ♀ ▶- $

Progestins

hydroxyprogesterone caproate (*Hylutin*): Amenorrhea, dysfunctional uterine bleeding, metorrhagia: 375mg IM. Production of secretory endometrium and desquamation: 125-250mg IM on 10th day of the cycle, repeat q7days until suppression no longer desired. ▶L ♀X ▶? $

medroxyprogesterone acetate (*Provera, Cycrin, Amen, Curretab*): HRT: 10mg PO qd for last 12 days of month, or 2.5-5mg PO qd continuously. Secondary amenorrhea: 5-10mg PO qd X 5-10 days. Abnormal uterine bleeding: 5-10mg PO qd X 5-10d. Endometrial hyperplasia: 10-30mg PO qd. [Generic/Trade: Tabs 2.5, 5, & 10mg, scored.] ▶L ♀X ▶+ $

medroxyprogesterone acetate (injectable contraceptive) (*Depo-Provera*): Contraception: 150mg IM q13 weeks. ▶L ♀X ▶+ $

megestrol (*Megace*): Endometrial hyperplasia: 40-160mg PO qd X 3-4 mo. AIDS anorexia: 800mg susp PO qd. [Trade: Tabs 20 & 40mg; Susp 40mg/ml in 237ml (pints).] ▶L ♀D ▶? $$$$$

norethindrone (*Aygestin, Norlutate*): Amenorrhea, abnormal uterine bleeding: 2.5-10mg PO qd x5-10d during the second ½ of cycle. Endometriosis: 5mg PO qd X 2 weeks; increase by 2.5mg q 2 weeks to 15mg. [Trade: Tabs 5mg, scored.] ▶L ♀D ◗? $

progesterone, micronized (*Prometrium*): HRT: 200mg PO hs 12 days per month or 100 mg hs continuously. Secondary amenorrhea: 400mg PO hs X 10 days. Contains peanut oil; avoid in peanut allergy. [Caps 100 & 200mg.] ▶L ♀X ◗+ $

Selective Estrogen Receptor Modulators

raloxifene (*Evista*): Osteoporosis prevention/treatment: 60mg PO qd. [Trade: Tabs 60mg.] ▶L ♀X ◗- $$$

tamoxifen (*Nolvadex, Tamone*): Breast cancer prevention: 20mg PO qd X 5 years. [Generic/Trade: Tabs 10 & 20mg.] ▶L ♀D ◗- $$$

Tocolytics

indomethacin (*Indocin, Indocid*): Pretem labor: initial 50-100mg PO/PR followed by 25mg PO/PR q6-12h up to 48 hrs. [Generic/Trade: Immediate release Caps 25 & 50mg; Trade; Oral Susp 25mg/5ml; supp 50mg .] ▶L ♀? ◗- $

magnesium sulfate: Eclampsia: 1-4g IV over 2-4 min. Drip: 5g in 250ml D5W (20mg/ml), 2g/h = 100ml/h. Preterm labor: 6g IV over 20 minutes, then 2-3g/h titrated to decrease contractions. Monitor respirations & reflexes. If needed, may reverse effects with calcium gluconate 1 g IV. ▶K ♀A ◗+ $

nifedipine (*Procardia, Adalat, Procardia XL, Adalat CC*): Preterm labor: loading dose: 10mg PO q20-30 min if contractions persist, up to 40mg within the first 1h. Maintenance dose: 10-20mg PO q4-6h or 60-160mg extended release PO qd. [Generic/Trade: immed release Caps 10 & 20mg. Ext release tabs 30,60,90mg.] ▶L ♀C ◗- $

ritodrine (*Yutopar*): Start 0.05mg/min IV infusion; increase by 0.05mg/min q10min until desired result; usual range 0.15-0.35mg/min for at least 12h until contractions cease. Infusion: 150mg in 500ml D5W (0.3mg/ml), 50mcg/min = 10ml/h. ▶K ♀B ◗- $$$$

terbutaline (*Brethine, Bricanyl*): Preterm labor: 0.25mg SC q30 min up to 1mg per four hrs. Infusion: 2.5-10mcg/min IV, gradually increased to effective max doses of 17.5-30mcg/minute. 2.5-5mg PO q4-6h maintenance until term. Tachycardia common. [Tabs 2.5, 5mg.] ▶L ♀B ◗+ $

Uterotonics (post-partum bleeding)

carboprost (*Hemabate, 15-methyl-prostaglandin F2 alpha*): 250 mcg deep IM. ▶LK ♀C ◗? $$

methylergonovine (*Methergine*): 0.2mg IM/PO tid-qid prn. [Trade: Tabs 0.2mg.] ▶LK ♀C ◗? $

oxytocin (*Pitocin*): 10 units IM or 10-40 units in 1000ml NS IV. ▶LK ♀? ◗? $

Vaginal Preparations (See also STD/vaginitis table in antimicrobial section)

butoconazole (*Femstat 3, Gynazole-1*): Vulvovaginal candidiasis: Femstat 3: 1 applicatorful hs x3-6d; Gynazole-1: 1 applicatorful intravaginally hs x1. [OTC: Trade (Femstat 3): 2% vaginal cream in 5g pre-filled applicators (3s) & 20g tube with applicators; Rx: Trade (Gynazole-1): 2% vaginal cream in 5g pre-filled applicator.] ▶LK ♀C ◗? $

clindamycin phosphate (*Cleocin, Dalacin*): Bacterial vaginosis: 1 applicatorful cream hs x 7d or one supp qhs x 3d. [Trade: 2% vaginal cream in 21 g tube with 3 disposable applicators or 40g tube with 7 applicators. Vag supp 100 (3).] ▶L ♀B ◗+ $$

clotrimazole (*Mycelex, Gyne-Lotrimin, Femcare, Sweet'n fresh, Canestin*): Vulvovaginal candidiasis: 1 applicatorful 1% cream hs X 7 days; 1 applicatorful 2% cream hs X 3 days; 1 vag tab 100mg hs X 7days; 1 vag tab 200mg hs X 3days or 500mg vaginal tablet hs single-dose. [OTC: Generic/Trade: 1% vaginal cream with applicator (some pre-filled); Trade (Gyne-Lotrimin-3): 2% vaginal cream with applicator (21g); Generic/Trade: vaginal Tabs 100mg (7); Trade: vaginal Tabs 200mg (3) & 500mg (1) with applicators; 1% topical cream in some combination packs.] ▶LK ♀B ▶? $

estradiol vaginal ring (*Estring*): Insert and replace after 90 days. [2 mg] ▶L ♀X ▶- $

estradiol vaginal tablet (*Vagifem*): One tablet vaginally qd x2 wks, then one tab 2x/week. [Trade: Vaginal tab: 25mcg in single-use applicators, 15/pack.] ▶L ♀X ▶- $$

estrogen cream (*Premarin, Estrace, Ogen, Ortho Dienestrol*): Atrophic vaginitis: Premarin: 0.5-2g qd 3 wks of month. Estrace: 2-4 g qd x 2 weeks, then reduce. Ogen: 2-4g qd 3 wks of month. Ortho Dienestrol: 1-2 applicatorsful qd for 1-2 weeks, then reduce. [Trade: Vaginal cream. Premarin: 0.625mg conjugated estrogens/g in 42.5g with or w/o calibrated applicator. Estrace: 0.1mg estradiol/g in 42.5g w/calibrated applicator. Ogen: 1.5mg estropipate/g in 42.5g with calibrated applicator. Ortho Dienestrol: 0.01% dienestrol in 78g with or w/o applicator.] ▶L ♀X ▶? $$

metronidazole (*MetroGel-Vaginal*): Bacterial vaginosis: 1 applicatorful hs or bid X 5 days. [Trade: 0.75% gel in 70g tube with applicator.] ▶LK ♀B ▶? $$

miconazole (*Monistat-3, Monistat-7, Monistat Dual Pak, Femizol, M-Zole, Micozole, Monazole*): Vulvovaginal candidiasis: 1 applicatorful hs X 7 days; 100mg vag supp hs x7d; 200mg vag supp hs x3d; 1200mg vaginal insert hs x1. [OTC: Generic/Trade: 2% vag cream in 45g; OTC: Trade: vag supp 100mg; Rx: Trade: Monistat Dual Pak ($$): 1200mg soft gel vag insert plus 2% miconazole cream for external use.] ▶LK ♀+ ▶? $

nystatin (*Mycostatin, Candistatin*): Vulvovaginal candidiasis: 1 vag tab hs X 14 days. [Generic/Trade: Vaginal Tabs 100,000 units in 15s & 30s] ▶Not metabolized ♀A ▶? $

progesterone gel (*Crinone*): Specialized dosing for infertility. [Trade: Vaginal gel 4% (45mg), 8% (90mg) in single use applicator.] ▶L ♀D ▶+ $$$

terconazole (*Terazol*): Vulvovaginal candidiasis: 1 applicatorful of 0.4% cream hs x 7 days; 1 applicatorful of 0.8% cream hs x 3 days; 80mg vag supp hs x3d. [Trade: Vag cream 0.4% in 45g tube; vag cream 0.8% in 20g tube; vag supp 80mg] ▶LK ♀C ▶- $$

tioconazole (*Monistat-1, Vagistat-1, Gynecure*): Vulvovaginal candidiasis: 1 applicatorful of 6.5% ointment intravaginally hs single-dose. [OTC: Trade: Vaginal ointment: 6.5% (300 mg) in 4.6g prefilled single-dose applicator.] ▶Not absorbed ♀C ▶- $

Other OB/GYN Agents

betamethasone (*Celestone*): Fetal lung maturation, maternal antepartum: 12mg IM q24h x 2 doses. ▶L ♀C ▶- $$

clomiphene (*Clomid, Serophene*): Specialized dosing for ovulation induction. [Generic/Trade: Tabs 50mg, scored.] ▶L ♀D ▶? $$

clonidine (*Catapres, Catapres-TTS*): Menopausal flushing: 0.1-0.4mg/day PO divided bid/tid. Transdermal system 0.1mg/day, 1 patch qweek. [Generic/Trade: Tabs 0.1, 0.2, & 0.3mg. Trade: Transdermal patch: 0.1, 0.2, & 0.3mg/24 hours.] ▶KL ♀C ▶? $

danazol (*Danocrine*): Endometriosis: start 400mg PO bid, then titrate downward to maintain amenorrhea X 3-6 months. Fibrocystic breast disease: 100-200mg PO bid x 4-6 months. [Generic/Trade: Caps 50, 100, 200mg.] ▶L ♀X ▶- $$$$

dexamethasone (*Decadron*): Fetal lung maturation, maternal antepartum: 6mg IM q12h x 4 doses. ▶L ♀C ▶- $

fluconazole (*Diflucan*): Vaginal candidiasis: 150mg PO single dose. [Trade: Tabs 50, 100, 150, & 200mg; Susp 10mg/ml & 40mg/ml.] ▶K ♀C ▶- $

gonadotropins (menotropins) (*FSH/LH, Pergonal, Humegon, Repronex*): Specialized dosing for ovulation induction. ▶L ♀X ▶? $$$$$

Premesis-Rx (B6/folic acid/B12/calcium carbonate): Pregnancy-induced nausea: 1 tab PO qd. [Trade: Tabs 75 mg vitamin B6 (pyridoxine), sustained-release, 12 mcg vitamin B12 (cyanocobalamin), 1 mg folic acid, and 200 mg calcium carb] ▶L ♀A ▶+ $

RHO immune globulin (*RhoGAM, Gamulin Rh, HypRho-D, Mini-Gamulin Rh, HypRho-D Mini-Dose*): 1 vial (300mcg) IM within 72h if mother Rh-. ▶L ♀C ▶? $$$$

ONCOLOGY – Variable dosages. **Alkylating agents**: busulfan (*Myleran*), carboplatin (*Paraplatin*), carmustine (*BCNU, BiCNU, Gliadel*), chlorambucil (*Leukeran*), cisplatin (*Platinol*), cyclophosphamide (*Cytoxan, Neosar*), dacarbazine (*DTIC-Dome*), ifosfamide (*Ifex*), lomustine (*CCNU, CeeNu*), mechlorethamine (*Mustargen*), melphalan (*Alkeran*), procarbazine (*Matulane*), streptozocin (*Zanosar*), temozolomide (*Temodar*), thiotepa (*Thioplex*). **Antibiotics**: bleomycin (*Blenoxane*), dactinomycin (*Cosmegen*), daunorubicin (*DaunoXome, Cerubidine*), doxorubicin (*Adriamycin, Rubex, Doxil*), epirubicin (*Ellence*), idarubicin (*Idamycin*), mitomycin (*Mutamycin*), mitoxantrone (*Novantrone*), plicamycin (*mithramycin, Mithracin*), valrubicin (*Valstar*). **Antimetabolites**: capecitabine (*Xeloda*), cladribine (*Leustatin*), cytarabine (*ARA-C, Cytosar-U*), floxuridine (*FUDR*), fludarabine (*Fludara*), fluorouracil (*5-FU, Adrucil*), gemcitabine (*Gemzar*), hydroxyurea (*Hydrea, Doxia*), mercaptopurine (*6-MP, Purinethol*), methotrexate, pentostatin (*Nipent*), thioguanine. **Hormones**: anastrozole (*Arimidex*), bicalutamide (*Casodex*), estramustine (*Emcyt*), exemestane (*Aromasin*), flutamide (*Eulexin*), goserelin (*Zoladex*), irinotecan (*Camptosar*), letrozole (*Femara*), leuprolide (*Leupron*), nilutamide (*Nilandron, Anandron*), tamoxifen (*Nolvadex, Tamone*), topotecan (*Hycamtin*), toremifene (*Fareston*). **Immunomodulators**: aldesleukin (*Interleukin-2, Proleukin*), BCG (*Bacillus of Calmette & Guerin, TheraCys, Tice BCG Vaccine*), denileukin diftitox (*Ontak*), interferon alfa-2a (*Roferon-A*), interferon alfa-2b (*Intron A*), interferon alfa-n3 (*Alferon N*), rituximab (*Rituxan*), trastuzumab (*Herceptin*). **Mitotic Inhibitors**: docetaxel (*Taxotere*), etoposide (*VP-16, VePesid, Toposar*), paclitaxel (*Taxol*), teniposide (*Vumon*), vinblastine (*VLB, Velban*), vincristine (*VCR, Oncovin, Vincasar*), vinorelbine (*Navelbine*). **Radiopharmaceuticals**: samarium 153 (*Quadramet*), strontium-89 (*Metastron*). **Other**: altretamine (*Hexalen*), asparaginase (*Elspar*), levamisole (*Ergamisol*), mitotane (*Lysodren*), pegaspargase (*Oncaspar*), porfimer (*Photofrin*), tretinoin (*Vesanoid*).

OPHTHALMOLOGY

Antibacterials

bacitracin (*AK Tracin*): ointment q3-4h or bid-qid. [Generic/Trade: ointment 500 units/g.] ▶Not absorbed ♀C ▶? $

ciprofloxacin (*Ciloxan*): 1-2 gtt q1-6h or ½ inch ribbon ointment bid-tid. [Trade only: solution 0.3%, ointment 0.3%.] ▶LK ♀C ▶? $$

erythromycin (*Ilotycin, AK-Mycin*): ½ inch ribbon of ointment q3-4h or bid-qid. [Generic/Trade: ointment 0.5%.] ▶L ♀B ▶+ $

gentamicin (*Garamycin, Alcomicin*): 1-2 gtts q4h; ½ inch ribbon of oint bid-tid. [Generic/Trade: solution 0.3%, ointment 0.3%.] ▶K ♀C ▶? $

Neosporin Ointment (neomycin + bacitracin + polymyxin B): ½ inch ribbon of ointment q3-4h x 7-10 days. [Generic/Trade: ointment.] ▶K ♀C ◗? $

Neosporin solution (neomycin + polymyxin + gramicidin): 1-2 gtts q1-6h x 7-10 days. [Trage/generic: solution] ▶K ♀C ◗? $$

norfloxacin (*Chibroxin, Noroxin*): 1-2 gtts q2-6h. [Trade only: sol'n 0.3%.] ▶LK ♀C ◗? $

ofloxacin (*Ocuflox*): 1-2 gtts q1-6h x 7-10 days. [Trade only: sol'n 0.3%.] ▶LK ♀C ◗? $$

Polysporin (polymyxin B + bacitracin): ½ inch ribbon of ointment qd or q3-4 h x 7-10 days. [Generic/Trade: ointment.] ▶K ♀C ◗? $

Polytrim (polymyxin B + trimethoprim): 1 gtt q3-6h x 7-10d, max 6 gtts/day. [Trade only: solution.] ▶K ♀C ◗? $

sulfacetamide (*Sulamyd, Bleph-10, Sulf-10, Isopto Cetamide*): 1-2 gtts q2-6h x 7-10d or ½ inch ribbon of ointment q3-8h x 7-10d. [Generic/Trade: solution 1%, 10%, 15%, 30%. ointment 10%.] ▶K ♀C ◗- $

tobramycin (*Tobrex*): 1-2 gtts q1-4h or ½ inch ribbon of ointment q3-4h or bid-tid. [Generic/Trade: solution 0.3%. Trade only: ointment 0.3%.] ▶K ♀B ◗- $

Antiviral Agents

trifluridine (*Viroptic*): Herpes: 1 gtt q2-4h x 7-14d, max 9 gtts/day. [Trade only: solution 1%.] ▶Not absorbed ♀C ◗- $$$

vidarabine (*Vira-A*): ½ inch ribbon of ointment 5x daily (q3h) x5-7d. After re-epithelialization, ½ inch ribbon bid x 5-7 days. [Trade only: ointment 3%.] ▶Cornea ♀C ◗? $$$

Corticosteroids & Combinations

NOTE: Recommend that only ophthalmologists/optometrists prescribe due to infection risk.

Cortisporin (neomycin + polymyxin + hydrocortisone): 1-2 gtts or ½ inch ribbon of ointment q3-4h or more frequently prn. [Generic/Trade: susp, ointment.] ▶LK ♀C ◗? $

fluorometholone (*FML, FML Forte, Flarex*): 1-2 gtts q1-12h or ½ inch ribbon of ointment q4-24h. [Generic/Trade: susp 0.1%. Trade only: susp 0.25%. solution 0.1%, ointment 0.1%.] ▶L ♀C ◗? $$

loteprednol (*Alrex, Lotemax*): 1-2 gtts qid. [Trade only: susp 0.2% (Alrex), 0.5% (Lotemax).] ▶L ♀C ◗? $$

Maxitrol (dexamethasone + neomycin + polymyxin): 1-2 gtts q1-8h or ½ -1 inch ribbon of ointment qd-qid. [Generic/Trade: susp, ointment.] ▶KL ♀C ◗? $

prednisolone (*AK-Pred, Pred Forte, Pred Mild, Inflamase Forte*): 1 gtt q1-12h. [Generic/Trade: susp 0.12,0.125,1%, solution 0.125,1%.] ▶L ♀C ◗? $$

rimexolone (*Vexol*): 1-2 gtts q1-6h. [Trade only: susp 1%.] ▶L ♀C ◗? $$

TobraDex (tobramycin + dexamethasone): 1-2 gtts q2-6h or ½ inch ribbon of ointment bid-qid. [Trade only: ointment. Trade/generic: susp.] ▶L ♀C ◗? $$

Glaucoma Agents - Beta Blockers

NOTE: Use caution in cardiac conditions and asthma.

betaxolol (*Betoptic*): 1-2 gtts bid. [Trade only: susp 0.25%. Generic/Trade: solution 0.5%.] ▶LK ♀C ◗? $$

carteolol (*Ocupress*): 1 gtt bid. [Generic/Trade: solution 1%.] ▶KL ♀C ◗? $

levobunolol (*Betagan*): 1- 2 gtts qd-bid. [Generic/Trade: sol'n 0.25, 0.5%.] ▶? ♀C ◗- $

timolol (*Timoptic, Timoptic XE*): 1 gtt bid. Timoptic XE: 1 gtt qd. [Generic/Trade: solution 0.25%, 0.5%. gel forming solution 0.25, 0.5% (Timoptic XE).] ▶LK ♀C ◗+ $

Glaucoma Agents - Carbonic Anhydrase Inhibitors

NOTE: Sulfonamide derivatives; verify absence of sulfa allergy before prescribing.

acetazolamide (*Diamox*): Glaucoma: 250 mg PO qd-qid (immediate release) or 500 mg PO qd-bid (extended release). [Generic/Trade: Tabs 125, 250 mg. Trade only: extended release Caps 500 mg.] ▶LK ♀C ◗+ $$

brinzolamide (*Azopt*): 1 gtt tid. [Trade only: susp 1%.] ▶LK ♀C ◗? $

dorzolamide (*Trusopt*): 1 gtt tid. [Trade only: solution 2%.] ▶KL ♀C ◗ $$

Glaucoma Agents - Other

apraclonidine (*Iopidine*): 1-2 gtts tid. [Trade only: solution 0.5,1%.] ▶KL ♀C ◗? $$$

brimonidine (*Alphagan*): 1 gtt tid. [Trade only: solution 0.2%.] ▶L ♀B ◗? $$

Cosopt (dorzolamide + timolol): 1 gtt bid. [Trade only: solution (dorzolamide 2% + timolol 0.5%).] ▶LK ♀C ◗- $$

dipivefrin (*Propine*): 1 gtt q12h. [Generic/Trade: solution 0.1%.] ▶Eye, plasma ♀B ◗? $

echothiophate iodide (*Phospholine Iodide*): 1 gtt qd-bid. [Trade only: solution 0.03, 0.06, 0.125, 0.25%.] ▶? ♀C ◗- $$

latanoprost (*Xalatan*): 1 gtt hs. [Trade only: solution 0.005%.] ▶LK ♀C ◗? $$

pilocarpine (*Pilocar, Pilopine HS, Isopto Carpine, Diocarpine*): 1-2 gtts tid-qid or ½ inch ribbon of gel hs. [Generic/Trade: solution 0.5,1,2,3,4,6,8%. Trade only: 0.25,5,10%, gel 4%.] ▶Plasma ♀C ◗? $

Mydriatics & Cycloplegics

atropine (*Isopto Atropine*): 1-2 gtts before procedure or qd-qid, ointment before procedure or qd-tid. Cycloplegia lasts 5-10d; mydriasis lasts 7-14d. [Generic/Trade: solution 1,2%, ointment 1%. Trade only: solution 0.5%.] ▶K ♀C ◗+ $

cyclopentolate (*AK-Pentolate, Cyclogyl, Pentolair*): 1-2 gtts x 1-2 doses before procedure. Cycloplegia lasts 6-24h; mydriasis lasts 1d. [Generic/Trade: solution 1%. Trade only: 0.5,2%.] ▶? ♀C ◗? $

homatropine (*Isopto Homatropine*): 1-2 gtts before procedure or bid-tid. Cycloplegia & mydriasis lasts 1-3d. [Trade only: sol'n 2%. Generic/Trade: solution 5%.] ▶? ♀C ◗? $

phenylephrine (*Neo-Synephrine, Mydfrin, Relief*): 1-2 gtts before procedure or tid-qid with atropine. No cycloplegia; mydriasis lasts 5h. [Generic/Trade: solution 0.12, 2.5, 10%.] ▶Plasma ♀C ◗? $

tropicamide (*Mydriacyl*): 1-2 gtts before procedure. Cycloplegia & mydriasis lasts 6h. [Generic/Trade: solution 0.5, 1%.] ▶? ♀? ◗? $

Nonsteroidal Anti-Inflammatories

diclofenac (*Voltaren, Vofenal*): 1 gtt qid and/or before procedure. [Generic/Trade: solution 0.1%.] ▶L ♀B ◗? $$

ketorolac (*Acular*): 1 gtt qid. [Trade only: solution 0.5%.] ▶L ♀C ◗? $$$

Ocular Decongestants / Anti-Allergy

cromolyn sodium (*Crolom, Opticrom*): 1-2 gtts 4-6 times per day. [Generic/Trade: solution 4%.] ▶LK ♀B ◗? $$$

ketotifen (*Zaditor*): 1 gtt q8-12h. [Trade only: soln 0.025%.] ▶Not absorbed ♀C ◗? $$

levocabastine (*Livostin*): 1 gtt qid. [Trade only: susp 0.05%.] ▶? ♀C ◗? $$$

lodoxamide tromethamine (*Alomide*): 1-2 gtts qid. [Trade: sol'n 0.1%.] ▶K ♀B ◗? $$$

naphazoline (*Albalon, AK-Con, Vasocon, Naphcon, Allerest, Clear Eyes*): 1 gtt q3-4h prn up to qid. [Generic/Trade: solution 0.012, 0.02, 0.03, 0.1% .] ▶? ♀C ▶? $

Naphcon-A (naphazoline + pheniramine): 1-2 gtts bid-qid prn. [Generic/Trade: solution (0.025% naphazoline + 0.3% pheniramine).] ▶L ♀C ▶? $

nedocromil (*Alocril*): 1-2 gtts bid. [Trade only: solution 2%.] ▶L ♀B ▶? $$

olopatadine (*Patanol*): 1-2 gtts bid. [Trade only: solution 0.1%.] ▶K ♀C ▶? $$$

pemirolast (*Alamast*): 1-2 gtts qid. [Trade only: solution 0.1%.] ▶? ♀C ▶? ?

Other Ophthalmologic Agents

artificial tears (*Tears Naturale, Hypotears, Lacrilube*): 1-2 gtts tid-qid prn. [OTC solution.] ▶Not absorbed ♀A ▶+ $

proparacaine (*Ophthaine, Ophthetic*): Do not prescribe for unsupervised/prolonged use, corneal toxicity. 1-2 gtts before procedure. [Generic/Trade: sol'n 0.5%.] ▶L ♀C ▶? $

tetracaine (*Pontocaine*): Do not prescribe for unsupervised/prolonged use, corneal toxicity. 1-2 gtts or ½-1 inch ribbon of ointment before procedure. [Generic/Trade: sol'n 0.5%.] ▶Plasma ♀C ▶? $

PSYCHIATRY

Antidepressants - Selective Serotonin Reuptake Inhibitors (SSRIs)

citalopram (*Celexa*): Depression: Start 20 mg PO qd, max 60 mg/day. [Trade: Tabs 20, 40 mg. oral solution 10 mg/5ml.] ▶LK ♀C ▶- $$$

fluoxetine (*Prozac*): Depression & OCD: Start 20 mg PO q am, usual effective dose 20-40 mg/day, max 80 mg/day. Bulimia: 60 mg PO qd. [Trade: Caps 10, 20, 40 mg. Tabs 10 mg. oral solution 20 mg/ 5 ml.] ▶L ♀C ▶- $$$

fluvoxamine (*Luvox*): OCD: Start 50 mg PO hs, usual effective dose 100-300 mg/ day divided bid, max 300 mg/day. OCD and ≥8 yo: Start 25 mg PO hs, usual effective dose 50-200 mg/day divided bid, max 200 mg/day. Avoid with cisapride, diazepam, pimozide, and MAOIs; caution with benzodiazepines, TCAs, theophylline, and warfarin. [Trade: Tabs 25, 50, 100 mg.] ▶L ♀C ▶- $$$$

paroxetine (*Paxil*): Depression: Start 20 mg PO qam, usual effective dose 20-50 mg/day, max 50 mg/day. OCD/ panic disorder/ social phobia: Start 10-20 mg/day, usual effective dose 10-60 mg/day, max 60 mg/day. [Trade: Tabs 10, 20, 30, 40 mg. oral susp 10 mg/ 5 ml.] ▶LK ♀C ▶? $$$

sertraline (*Zoloft*): Depression/OCD: Start 50 mg PO qd, usual effective dose 50-200 mg/d, max 200 mg/d. Panic disorder/ Posttraumatic stress disorder: Start 25 mg PO qd, max 200 mg/d. [Trade: Tabs 25,50,100 mg. oral conc 20 mg/ml.] ▶LK ♀C ▶+ $$$

Antidepressants - Serotonin-Norepinephrine Reuptake Inhibitors (SNRIs)

amitriptyline (*Elavil, Vanatrip, Levate*): Start 25-100 mg PO hs, gradually increase to usual effective dose of 50-300 mg/d. Demethylated to nortriptyline. [Generic/Trade: Tabs 10, 25, 50, 75, 100, 150 mg.] ▶L ♀D ▶- $

clomipramine (*Anafranil*): Start 25 mg PO hs, gradually increase to usual effective dose of 150-250 mg/day, max 250 mg/day. Seizures. [Generic/Trade: Caps 25, 50, 75 mg.] ▶L ♀C ▶+ $$$

desipramine (*Norpramin*): Start 25 mg PO qd or in divided doses. Gradually increase to usual effective dose of 100-300 mg/d. [Generic/Trade: Tabs 10,25,50,75,100,150 mg.] ▶L ♀C ▶+ $

doxepin (*Sinequan, Zonalon, Triadapin*): Start 25 mg PO hs. Usual effective dose 75-300 mg/day. [Generic/Trade: Caps 10,25,50,75,100,150 mg. Oral concentrate10 mg/ml.] ▶L ♀C ▶- $

imipramine (*Tofranil, Impril*): Start 25 mg PO hs, gradually increase to usual effective dose 50-300 mg/d. Demethylated to desipramine. [Generic/Trade: Tabs 10, 25, 50 mg. Trade only: Caps 75, 100, 125, 150 mg.] ▶L ♀D ▶- $

nortriptyline (*Aventyl, Pamelor, Norventyl*): Start 25 mg PO qd- qid. Usual effective dose 50-150 mg/day. [Generic/Trade: Caps 10, 25, 50, 75 mg. Trade only: oral solution 10 mg/ 5 ml.] ▶L ♀D ▶+ $

venlafaxine (*Effexor, Effexor XR*): Depression/ anxiety: Start 37.5-75 mg PO qd (Effexor XR), max 225 mg/day; 75 mg/ day (Effexor) PO divided bid/tid, max 375 mg/day. Usual effective dose 150-225 mg/day [Trade: Caps, extended release 37.5, 75, 150 mg. Tabs 25, 37.5, 50, 75, 100 mg.] ▶K ♀C ▶? $$$$

Antidepressants - Other

bupropion (*Wellbutrin, Wellbutrin SR*): Depression: Start 100 mg PO bid, after 4-7 days can increase to 100 mg tid. Usual effective dose 300-450 mg/day. Max 150 mg/dose and 450 mg/day. Sustained release: Start 100-150 mg PO q am, after 4-7d may increase to 150 mg bid, max 400 mg/d. Last dose ≤5 pm. Contraindicated with anorexia, bulimia, seizures. Seizures in 0.4% at 300-450 mg/d. [Generic/Trade: Tabs 75,100 mg. Trade only: sust release Tabs 100, 150 mg (Wellbutrin SR).] ▶K ♀B ▶- $$$

mirtazapine (*Remeron*): Start 15 mg PO hs. Usual effective dose 15-45 mg/day. Agranulocytosis 0.1%. [Trade: Tabs 15, 30, 45 mg.] ▶LK ♀C ▶? $$$

nefazodone (*Serzone*): Start 100 mg PO bid, usual effective dose 150-300 mg PO bid, max 600 mg/day. Avoid with cisapride, MAOIs, or triazolam. [Trade: Tabs 50, 100, 150, 200, 250 mg.] ▶L ♀C ▶? $$$

trazodone (*Desyrel, Trazorel*): Start 50-150 mg/day PO in divided doses. Usual effective dose is 400-600 mg/day in divided doses. [Generic/Trade: Tabs 50, 100, 150. Trade only: Tabs 300 mg.] ▶L ♀C ▶- $$

Antimanic (Bimodal) Agents

carbamazepine (*Tegretol, Tegretol XR, Carbatrol, Epitol, Mazepine*): Mania: 200 mg PO qd-bid, increase by 200 mg/ day q2-4 days. Mean effective dose = 1,000 mg/day. Aplastic anemia. [Generic/Trade: Tabs 200 mg. chewable Tabs 100 mg. Trade only: extended release Tabs 100, 200, 300, 400 mg. susp 100 mg/ 5 ml.] ▶LK ♀D ▶+ $

lithium (*Eskalith, Lithane, Lithobid, Lithonate, Carbolith, Duralith*): Start 300 mg PO bid, usual effective dose 900-1800 mg/d. 300 mg = 8 mEq or mmol. Steady state in 5d. Trough levels for acute mania 1.0-1.5 mEq/L, maintenance 0.6-1.2 mEq/L. Dose increase of 300 mg/d raises level by ~0.2 mEq/L. Monitor renal, thyroid function. Diuretics & ACE inhibitors increase levels. Avoid dehydration, salt restriction & many NSAIDS (ASA & sulindac OK). [Generic/Trade: Caps 150,300,600 mg. Tabs 300 mg. Trade only: extended release Tabs 300, 450 mg. syrup 300 mg/ 5ml.] ▶K ♀D ▶- $

valproic acid (*Depakene, Depakote, Depacon, Deproic, Epiject, Epival*): Mania: 250 mg PO tid. Hepatotoxicity, drug interactions, reduce dose in elderly. [Generic/Trade: Caps (Depakene) 250 mg. syrup (Depakene) 250 mg/ 5 ml. Trade only: sprinkle Caps (Depakote) 125 mg. Tabs, delayed release (Depakote) 125, 250, 500 mg.] ▶L ♀D ▶+ $

Antipsychotics - Atypical - Serotonin Dopamine Receptor Antagonists

clozapine (*Clozaril*): Start 12.5 mg PO qd-bid. Usual effective dose 300-450 mg/day divided bid. Max 900 mg/day. Agranulocytosis 1-2%; check WBC counts q week x 6 months, then q2 weeks. [Generic/Trade: Tabs 25, 100 mg.] ▶L ♀B ▶- $$$$$

olanzapine (*Zyprexa*): Start 5-10 mg PO qd; usual effective dose 10-15 mg/day. Bipolar mania: Start 10-15 mg PO qd; usual effective dose 5-20 mg/day. Max 20 mg/day. [Trade: Tabs 2.5, 5, 7.5, 10, 15 mg.] ▶L ♀C ▶- $$$$$

quetiapine (*Seroquel*): Start 25 mg PO bid. Usual effective dose 150-750 mg/day. Eye exam for cataracts recommended q 6 months. [Trade: Tabs 25, 100, 200 mg.] ▶LK ♀C ▶- $$$$$

risperidone (*Risperdal*): Start 1 mg PO bid (0.5 mg/dose in the elderly), slowly increase to usual effective dose of 4-8 mg/day divided qd-bid. Max 16 mg/day. Low EPS risk <10 mg/day. [Trade: Tabs 0.25,0.5,1,2,3,4 mg. oral sol'n 1 mg/ml] ▶LK ♀C ▶- $$$$$

Antipsychotics - D2 Antagonists

chlorpromazine (*Thorazine, Chlorpromanyl*): Start 10-50 mg PO/IM bid/tid, usual dose 300-800 mg/d. [Generic/Trade: Tabs 10, 25, 50, 100, 200 mg. oral concentrate 30 mg/ml, 100 mg/ml. Trade only: sustained release Caps 30, 75, 150 mg. syrup 10 mg/5ml. supp 25, 100 mg.] ▶LK ♀C ▶- $

fluphenazine (*Prolixin, Permitil, Modecate, Moditen*): 1.25- 10 mg/ day IM divided q6-8h. Start 0.5- 10 mg/day PO divided q6-8h. Usual effective dose 1-20 mg/day. 2 mg = 100 CPZ. Depot (fluphenazine decanoate/ enanthate): 12.5-25 mg IM/SC q3 weeks = 10-20 mg/day PO fluphenazine. [Generic/Trade: Tabs 1, 2.5, 5, 10 mg. elixir 2.5 mg/5ml. oral concentrate 5 mg/ml.] ▶LK ♀C ▶? $$

haloperidol (*Haldol, Peridol*): 2-5 mg IM. Start 0.5- 5 mg PO bid-tid, usual effective dose 6-20 mg/day. Therapeutic range 2-15 ng/ml. 2mg = 100 mg CPZ. Depot haloperidol (haloperidol decanoate): 100-200 mg IM q4 weeks = 10 mg/day oral haloperidol. [Generic/ Trade: Tabs 0.5, 1, 2, 5, 10, 20 mg. oral concentrate 2 mg/ml.] ▶LK ♀C ▶- $

loxapine (*Loxitane, Loxapac*): 12.5-50 mg IM q4-12h. Start 10 mg PO bid, usual effective dose 60-100 mg/day. Max 250 mg/d. 15 mg = 100 mg CPZ. [Generic/Trade: Caps 5, 10, 25, 50 mg. Trade only: oral concentrate 25 mg/ml.] ▶LK ♀C ▶- $$$

molindone (*Moban*): Start 50- 75 mg/ day PO divided tid- qid, usual effective dose 50-100 mg/day. Max 225 mg/day. 10 mg = 100 mg CPZ. [Trade: Tabs 5, 10, 25, 50, 100 mg. oral concentrate 20 mg/ml.] ▶LK ♀C ▶? $$$$$

thioridazine (*Mellaril*): Start 50-100 mg PO tid, usual dose 200-800 mg/day. Not first-line due to QTc prolongation, torsade de pointes, sudden death. Contraindicated with SSRIs, propranolol, pindolol. Monitor baseline ECG and K+. Pigmentary retinopathy with doses> 800 mg/d. [Generic/Trade: Tabs 10,15,25,50,100,150,200 mg. oral conc 30,100 mg/ml. Trade only: oral susp 25, 100 mg/5ml.] ▶LK ♀C ▶? $

Anxiolytics / Hypnotics - Benzodiazepines

alprazolam (*Xanax*): 0.25-0.5 mg PO bid-tid. Half-life 12h. Multiple drug interactions. [Generic/Trade: Tabs 0.25, 0.5, 1, 2 mg. Trade only: oral concentrate 1 mg/ml.] ▶LK ♀D ▶- ©IV $

chlordiazepoxide (*Librium*): Anxiety: 5-25 mg PO or 25-50 mg IM/IV tid/qid. Acute alcohol withdrawal: 50-100 mg PO/IM/IV, repeat q3-4h prn up to 300 mg/day. Half-life 5-30 h. [Generic/Trade: Caps 5, 10, 25 mg.] ▶LK ♀D ▶- ©IV $

clonazepam (*Klonopin, Rivotril, Clonapam*): Start 0.25-0.5 mg PO tid, max 4 mg/day. Half-life 18- 50 h. [Generic/Trade: Tabs 0.5, 1, 2 mg.] ▶LK ♀D ▶? ©IV $$

diazepam (*Valium, Vivol, E Pam*): Anxiety: 2-10 mg PO bid/qid. Half-life 20-80h. [Generic/Trade: Tabs 2, 5, 10 mg. oral solution 5 mg/ 5 ml. Trade only: oral concentrate (Intensol) 5 mg/ml.] ▶LK ♀D ▶- ©IV $

estazolam (*ProSom*): 1-2 mg PO hs. [Generic/Trade: Tabs 1, 2 mg.] ▶LK ♀X ▶- ©IV $$

flurazepam (*Dalmane, Somnol, Som Pam*): 15-30 mg PO hs. Half life 70-90h [Generic/Trade: Caps 15, 30 mg.] ▶LK ♀X ▶- ©IV $

lorazepam (*Ativan*): 0.5-2 mg IV/IM/PO q6-8h, max 10 mg/d. Half-life 10-20h. [Generic/ Trade: Tabs 0.5, 1, 2 mg. Trade only: oral concentrate 2 mg/ml.] ▶LK ♀D ▶- ©IV $$$

midazolam (*Versed*): Sedation/anxiolysis dose, see anesthesia section. ▶LK♀D▶-©IV $

oxazepam (*Serax, Zapex, Novoxapam, Oxpam*): 10-30 mg PO tid/qid. Half-life 8h. [Generic/Trade: Caps 10, 15, 30 mg.] ▶LK ♀D ▶- ©IV $$

temazepam (*Restoril*): 7.5-30 mg PO hs. Half-life 8-25h. [Generic/Trade: Caps 7.5, 15, 30 mg.] ▶LK ♀X ▶- ©IV $

triazolam (*Halcion*): 0.125-0.5 mg PO hs. 0.125 mg/day in elderly. Half-life 2-3h. [Generic/Trade: Tabs 0.125, 0.25 mg.] ▶LK ♀X ▶- ©IV $

Anxiolytics / Hypnotics - Other

buspirone (*BuSpar, Buspirex, Bustab*): Anxiety: Start 15 mg "dividose" daily (7.5 mg PO bid), usual effective dose 30 mg/day. Max 60 mg/day. [Trade: Tabs 5, 10 mg. dividose tablet 15,30 mg (scored to be easily bisected or trisected).] ▶K ♀B ▶- $$$

chloral hydrate (*Somnote, Aquachloral Supprettes*): 25-50 mg/kg/day up to 1000 mg PO/PR. Many physicians use higher than recommended doses in children (eg, 75 mg/kg). [Generic/Trade: Caps 500 mg. syrup 500 mg/ 5 ml. supp 500 mg. Trade only: supp: 324, 648 mg.] ▶LK ♀C ▶+ ©IV $

diphenhydramine (*Benadryl, Banaril, Allermax, Diphen, Dytuss, Sominex, Truxadryl, Tusstat, Allerdryl, Allernix*): Insomnia: 25-50 mg PO hs. Peds ≥12 yo: 50 mg PO hs. EPS: 25-50 mg PO tid-qid or 10-50 mg IV/IM tid-qid. [OTC/Generic/Trade: Tabs 25,50 mg. OTC/Trade: chew Tabs 12.5 mg. OTC/ Generic/Trade: Caps 25,50 mg. Sol'n 12.5 mg/5ml.] ▶LK ♀B(- in 1st trimester) ▶- $

pentobarbital (*Nembutal, Nova Rectal*): 20-150 mg PO/IV/IM/PR tid/qid. Peds: 2-6 mg/kg/day. [Trade: Caps 50, 100 mg. supp 60, 200 mg.] ▶LK ♀D ▶? ©II $

zaleplon (*Sonata*): 5-10 mg PO hs prn, max 20 mg. Do not use for benzodiazepine or ethanol withdrawal. [Trade: Caps 5, 10 mg.] ▶L ♀C ▶- ©IV $$$

zolpidem (*Ambien*): 5-10 mg PO hs. Do not use for benzodiazepine or ethanol withdrawal. [Trade: Tabs 5, 10 mg.] ▶L ♀B ▶+ ©IV $$$

Drug Dependence Therapy

bupropion (*Zyban*): Start 150 mg PO qam x 3d, then increase to 150 mg PO bid x 7-12 wks. Max dose 150 mg PO bid. Last dose no later than 5 pm. Contraindicated with seizures, bulimia, anorexia. Seizures in 0.4% at 300-450 mg/day. [Trade: sustained release Tabs 150 mg.] ▶K ♀B ▶- $$$

clonidine (*Catapres, Catapres TTS, Dixarit*): Opioid/ nicotine withdrawal, alcohol withdrawal adjunct (not FDA approved): 0.1- 0.3 mg PO tid- qid. Transdermal Therapeutic System (TTS) is designed for seven day use so that a TTS-1 delivers 0.1mg/day x 7 days. May supplement first dose of TTS with oral x 2-3 days while therapeutic level is achieved. [Generic/Trade: Tabs 0.1, 0.2, 0.3 mg. Trade only: patch TTS-1, TTS- 2, TTS- 3.] ▶LK ♀C ▶? $

disulfiram (*Antabuse*): Sobriety: 125-500 mg PO qd. Patient must abstain from any alcohol for ≥12 hours before using. Metronidazole and alcohol in any form (cough syrups, tonics, etc.) contraindicated. [Generic/Trade: Tabs 250, 500 mg.] ▸L ♀C ▸? $

methadone (*Dolophine, Methadose*): Narcotic dependence: 15-60 mg PO q6-8h. Treatment >3 wks is maintenance and only permitted in approved treatment programs. [Generic/Trade: Tabs 5, 10, 40 mg. oral solution 5 & 10 mg/5ml. oral concentrate 10 mg/ml.] ▸L ♀B ▸? ©II $$

naltrexone (*ReVia*): Alcohol/narcotic dependence: 25-50 mg PO qd. Avoid if recent ingestion of opioids (past 7-10 days). Hepatotoxicity with higher than approved doses. [Generic/Trade: Tabs 50 mg.] ▸LK ♀C ▸? $$$$

nicotine gum (*Nicorette, Nicorette DS*): Smoking cessation: Gradually taper 1 piece q1-2h x 6 weeks, 1 piece q2-4h x 3 weeks, then 1 piece q4-8h x 3 weeks, max 30 pieces/day of 2 mg or 24 pieces/ day of 4 mg. Use Nicorette DS 4 mg/piece in high cigarette use (> 24 cigarettes/day). [OTC/Trade: gum 2, 4 mg.] ▸LK ♀X ▸- $$$$$

nicotine inhalation system (*Nicotrol Inhaler*): 6-16 cartridges/day x 12 wks [Trade: inhaler 10 mg/cartridge (4 mg nicotine delivered), 42 cartridges/box.] ▸LK ♀D ▸- $$$$$

nicotine nasal spray (*Nicotrol NS*): Smoking cessation:1-2 doses each hour, with each dose = 2 sprays, one in each nostril (1 spray = 0.5 mg nicotine). Minimum recommended: 8 doses/day, max 40 doses/day. [Trade: nasal solution 10 mg/ml (0.5 mg/ inhalation); 10 ml bottles.] ▸LK ♀D ▸- $$$$$

nicotine patches (*Habitrol, Nicoderm, Nicotrol*): Smoking cessation: Start one patch (14-22 mg) qd, taper after 6 wks. Ensure patient has stopped smoking. [OTC/Rx/ Generic/Trade: patches 11, 22 mg/ 24 hours. 7, 14, 21 mg/ 24 hours (Habitrol & Nicoderm). OTC/Trade: 15 mg/ 16 hours (Nicotrol).] ▸LK ♀D ▸- $$$

Sympathomimetics / Stimulants / Anorexiants

Adderall (dextroamphetamine & racemic amphetamine): ADHD: Start 2.5 mg (3-5 yo) or 5 mg (≥6 yo) PO qd-bid, increase by 2.5-5 mg every week, max 40 mg/d. Narcolepsy: Start 5-10 mg PO q am, increase by 5-10 mg q week, max 60 mg/d. Avoid evening doses. Monitor growth and use drug holidays when appropriate. [Trade: Tabs 5, 10, 20, 30 mg.] ▸L ♀C ▸- ©II $$

caffeine (*NoDoz, Vivarin, Caffedrine, Stay Awake, Quick-Pep*): 100-200 mg PO q3-4h prn. [OTC/Generic/Trade: Tabs 200 mg. OTC/Trade: extended release Tabs 200 mg.] ▸L ♀B ▸? $

dextroamphetamine (*Dexedrine, Dextrostat*): Narcolepsy/ ADHD: 2.5-10 mg PO qam or bid-tid or 10-15 mg PO qd (sustained release), max 60 mg/d. Avoid evening doses. Monitor growth and use drug holidays when appropriate. [Trade: Tabs 5, 10 mg. Caps, sustained release 5, 10, 15 mg.] ▸L ♀C ▸- ©II $$

methylphenidate (*Ritalin, Methylin, Methylin ER, Metadate ER, Riphenidate, Concerta*): Narcolepsy/ADHD: 5-10 mg PO bid/tid or 20 mg PO qam (sust'd release), max 60 mg/d. Or 18-36 mg PO qam (ext'd release), max 54 mg/d. Avoid pm doses. Monitor growth & use drug holidays prn. [Generic/Trade: tablets 5, 10, 20 mg. sustained release tablets 10, 20 mg. extended release tablets 18,36 mg] ▸LK ♀C ▸? ©II $

modafinil (*Provigil, Alertec*): 200 mg PO qam. [Trade: Tabs 100, 200 mg.] ▸L ♀C ▸? ©IV $$$$

phentermine (*Adipex-P, Ionamin, Phentride, Phentercot, Teramine, Pro-Fast, OBY-Trim*): 8 mg PO tid or 15-37.5 mg/day q am or 10-14 hours before retiring. For short-term use. [Generic/Trade: Caps 15, 18.75, 30, 37.5 mg. Tabs 8, 37.5 mg. Trade only: extended release Caps 15, 30 mg (Ionamin).] ▸KL ♀C ▸- ©IV $

sibutramine (*Meridia*): Start 10 mg PO q am, max 15 mg/d. Monitor pulse and BP. [Trade: Caps 5, 10, 15 mg.] ▶KL ♀C ◗- ©IV $$$

Other Agents

benztropine (*Cogentin, Bensylate*): EPS: 1-4 mg PO/IM/IV qd-bid. [Generic/Trade: Tabs 0.5, 1, 2 mg.] ▶LK ♀C ◗? $

clonidine (*Catapres, Dixarit*): ADHD (peds): 5 mcg/kg/day PO x 8 wks. [Generic/Trade: Tabs 0.1,0.2,0.3 mg. Trade: patch TTS-1, TTS-2, TTS-3.] ▶LK ♀C ◗? $

fluoxetine (*Sarafem*): Premenstrual Dysphoric Disorder (PMDD): 20 mg PO qd. [Trade: Caps 10, 20 mg.] ▶L ♀C ◗- $$$

guanfacine (*Tenex*): ADHD (unapproved peds): Start 0.5 mg PO qd, titrate by 0.5 mg q3-4 days as tolerated to 0.5 mg PO tid. [Generic/Trade: Tabs 1, 2 mg.] ▶K ♀B ◗? $$

PULMONARY

Beta Agonists

albuterol (*Ventolin, Proventil, Volmax, Alromir, Asmavent, Ventodisk*): MDI 2 puffs q4-6h prn. 0.5ml of 0.5% sol'n (2.5mg) nebulized tid/qid. One 3ml unit dose (0.083%) nebulized tid-qid. Caps for inhalation 200-400mcg q4-6h. 2-4mg PO tid/qid or extended release 4-8mg PO q12h up to 16mg PO q12h. Children 2-6 yo: 0.1-0.2 mg/kg/dose PO tid up to 4mg tid; 6-12 yo: 2-4mg. [Generic/Trade: MDI 90mcg/actuation, 200/canister; sol'n for inhalation 0.5% (5mg/ml) in 20ml; nebules for inhalation 3ml unit dose (0.083%); Caps for inhalation 200mcg microfine in 24s & 96s w/ Rotahaler; Tabs 2 & 4mg; syrup 2mg/5ml; Trade: extended release tabs 4 & 8mg.] ▶L ♀C ◗? $

bitoltorol (*Tornalate*): MDI: 2 puffs q8h. Sol'n for inh 0.5-1ml tid/qid via intermittent flow or 1.25ml tid/qid via continuous flow. [Trade: MDI 0.37 mg/actuation, ~300/canister; sol'n for inhalation 0.2% (2mg/ml) with dropper.] ▶L ♀C ◗? $$

levalbuterol (*Xopenex*): 0.63-1.25mg nebulized q6-8h. [Trade: Sol'n for inhalation 0.63 & 1.25mg in 3ml unit-dose vials.] ▶L ♀C ◗? $$$$

metaproterenol (*Alupent, Metaprel, Pro-Meta*): MDI 2-3 puffs q3-4h: 0.2-0.3ml 5% sol'n nebulized q4h. 20mg PO tid/qid > 9 yo, 10mg PO tid-qid if 6-9 yo, 1.3-2.6mg/kg/d divided tid/qid if <6 yo. [Trade: MDI 0.65mg/actuation in 100 & 200/canister; Trade/Generic: sol'n for inhalation 0.4, 0.6% in unit-dose vials; 5% in unit-dose vials and 10 & 30ml with dropper; syrup 10mg/5ml; Generic: Tabs 10 & 20mg.] ▶L ♀C ◗? $$

pirbuterol (*Maxair, Maxair Autohaler*): 1-2 puffs q4-6h. [Trade: MDI 0.2mg/actuation, 300/canister, 400/canister (Autohaler).] ▶L ♀C ◗? $$

salmeterol (*Serevent, Serevent Diskus*): 2 puffs bid (Serevent). 1 puff bid (Serevent Diskus). Do not exceed these doses. Not for acute bronchospasm. [Trade: MDI: 25 mcg/actuation, 60 & 120/canister. Dry powder inhaler (Diskus): 50 mcg, 60 blisters.] ▶L ♀C ◗? $$$

terbutaline (*Brethine, Bricanyl*): 2.5-5mg PO q6h while awake in >12 yo. 0.25mg SC. [Trade: Tabs 2.5 & 5mg (Brethine scored).] ▶L ♀B ◗- $$

Combinations

Advair Diskus (fluticasone/salmeterol): Dosing unavailable at press time. [Trade: Dry powder inhaler: 100/50, 250/50, 500/50 mcg per actuation.] ▶L ♀C ◗? ?

Combivent (ipratropium/albuterol): 2 puffs qid, max 12 puffs/day. Contraindicated with soy & peanut allergy. [Trade: MDI: 18/90mcg/ actuation, 200/canister.] ▶L ♀C ◗? $$

WHAT COLOR IS WHAT INHALER? (Body then cap - Generics may differ)

Aerobid	grey/purple	*Flovent*	orange/peach	*Serevent*	teal/light teal
Aerobid-M	grey/green	*Intal*	white/blue	*Tilade*	white/white
Alupent	clear/blue	*Maxair*	blue/white	*Tornalate*	blue/blue
Atrovent	clear/green	*Maxair Autohaler*	white/white	*Vanceril*	pink/maroon
Azmacort	white/white			*Vanceril DS*	pink/maroon
Beclovent	cream/brown	*Proventil*	yellow/orange	*Ventolin*	light blue/navy
Combivent	clear/orange	*Pulmicort*	white/brown		

PREDICTED PEAK EXPIRATORY FLOW (liters/min) *Am Rev Resp Dis* 1963; 88:644

Age	Women *(height in inches)*					Men *(height in inches)*					Child	
(yrs)	55"	60"	65"	70"	75"	60"	65"	70"	75"	80"	*(height)*	
20	390	423	460	496	529	554	602	649	693	740	44"	160
30	380	413	448	483	516	532	577	522	664	710	46"	187
40	370	402	436	470	502	509	552	596	636	680	48"	214
50	360	391	424	457	488	486	527	569	607	649	50"	240
60	350	380	412	445	475	463	502	542	578	618	52"	267
70	340	369	400	432	461	440	477	515	550	587	54"	293

Inhaled Steroids (See Endocrine-Corticosteroids for oral steroids)

beclomethasone dipropionate (*Beclovent, Vanceril, Vanceril DS, Beclodisk*): Regular strength: 2 puffs tid/qid or 4 puffs bid. Double-strength: 2 puffs bid. [Trade: Beclovent, Vanceril MDI: 42mcg/ actuation, 80 & 200/canister. Vanceril DS MDI: 84 mcg/ actuation, 40 & 120/canister.] ▶L ♀C ▶? $$

budesonide (*Pulmicort Turbuhaler*): 1-2 puffs qd/bid. [Trade: Dry powder inhaler: 200mcg powder/actuation, 200/canister.] ▶L ♀C ▶? $$$$

flunisolide (*AeroBid, AeroBid-M*): 2-4 puffs bid. [Trade: MDI: 250mcg/actuation, 100/canister. AeroBid-M: menthol flavor.] ▶L ♀C ▶? $$$

fluticasone (*Flovent, Flovent Rotadisk*): 2-4 puffs bid. Dry powder inhaler: 1 puff bid, max 2 puffs bid. [Trade: MDI: 44, 110, 220mcg/actuation in 60 & 120/canister; dry powder inhaler (Rotadisk): 50, 100, & 250mcg/actuation, in 4 blisters containing 15 Rotadisks (total of 60 doses) with inhalation device.] ▶L ♀C ▶? $$$

triamcinolone acetonide (*Azmacort*): 2 puffs tid/qid or 4 puffs bid; max dose 16 puffs/ day. [Trade: MDI: 100mcg/actuation, 240/canister; built-in spacer.] ▶L ♀D ▶? $$$

Leukotriene Inhibitors

montelukast (*Singulair*): Adults: 10mg PO qpm. Children 2-5 yo: 4mg po q pm; 6-14 yo: 5mg PO qpm. [Trade: Tabs 4,5mg (chewable cherry flavor) & 10mg.] ▶L ♀B ▶? $$$

zafirlukast (*Accolate*): 20mg PO bid. Peds 7-11 yo, 10mg PO bid. Take at least 1h ac or 2h pc. Potentiates warfarin & theophylline. [Trade: Tabs 10, 20mg.] ▶L ♀B ▶- $$$

zileuton (*Zyflo*): 600mg PO qid. Hepatotoxicity, potentiates warfarin & theophylline [Trade: Tabs 600mg.] ▶L ♀C ▶? $$$$

Other Pulmonary Medications

acetylcysteine (*Mucomyst, Mucosil-10, Mucosil-20, Parvolex*): Mucolytic: 3-5ml of 20% or 6-10ml of 10% sol'n nebulized tid/qid. [Generic/Trade: Sol'n 10 & 20% in 4,10, & 30ml vials.] ▶L ♀B ▶? $$

cromolyn sodium (*Intal, Gastrocrom, Nalcrom*): 2-4 puffs qid or 20mg nebs qid. Oral concentrate: 200mg PO qid for adults, 100mg qid in children 2-12 yo. [Trade: MDI 800mcg/actuation, 112 & 200/canister; oral concentrate 5ml/100mg in 8 amps/foil pouch. Generic/Trade: Sol'n for nebs: 20mg/2ml.] ▶LK ♀B ▶? $$$

dexamethasone (*Decadron*): BPD preterm infants: 0.5mg/kg PO/IV divided q12h X 3 days, then taper. Croup: 0.15-0.6mg/kg PO or IM X 1. [Generic/Trade: Tabs 0.25, 0.5, 0.75, 1, 1.5, 2, 4, & 6mg, various scored; elixir: 0.5mg/5ml; oral sol'n: 0.5mg/5ml & 0.5mg/0.5ml.] ▶L ♀C ▶- $

dornase alfa (*Pulmozyme*): Cystic fibrosis: 2.5mg nebulized qd/bid. [Trade: Sol'n for inhalation: 1mg/ml in 2.5ml vials.] ▶L ♀B ▶? $$

epinephrine: Acute asthma & hypersensitivity reactions in adults: 0.1 to 0.3mg of 1:1,000 sol'n SC. Peds: 0.01mg/kg (up to 0.3mg) of 1:1,000 sol'n SC. Sustained release: 0.005mg/kg (up to 0.15mg) of 1:200 sol'n SC. [Sol'n for inj: 1:1,000 (1mg/ml in 1ml amps). Sust'd formulation (Sus-Phrine): 1:200 (5mg/ml) in 0.3ml amps or 5ml multi-dose vials. Injectable allergy kit in single-dose auto-injectors: Ana-Kit, Epipen, Epipen Jr.] ▶Plasma ♀C ▶- $

epinephrine racemic (*AsthmaNefrin, MicroNefrin, Nephron, S-2*): Severe croup: 0.05ml/kg/dose diluted to 3ml w/NS. [Trade: Sol'n for inhalation: 2.25% racepinephrine in 15 & 30ml.] ▶Plasma ♀C ▶- $

ipratropium (*Atrovent*): 2-3 puffs qid, or one 500mcg vial neb tid/qid. Contraindicated with soy/peanut allergy. [Trade: MDI: 18mcg/actuation, 200/canister; Generic/Trade: sol'n for nebulization: 0.02% (500mcg/vial) in unit dose vials.] ▶Lung ♀B ▶? $$

nedocromil (*Tilade*): 2 puffs qid. Reduce as tolerated [Trade: MDI: 1.75mg/actuation, 112/canister.] ▶L ♀B ▶? $$

theophylline (*Slo-Phyllin, Elixophyllin, Uni Dur, Uniphyl, Theo-24, Theo-Dur, Slo-bid*): 5-13mg/kg/d PO in divided doses. Max dose 900mg/d. Peds dosing variable. [Slo-Phyllin, Elixophyllin, various: Tabs 100,125,200,250,300mg, liquid 80mg/15ml, 150mg/15 ml; qd sust'd release Uni-Dur, Uniphyl, Theo-24: 100,200,300,400,600mg; bid sust'd release Theo-Dur, Slo-bid, various generics: 100, 200, 300 & 450mg.] ▶L ♀C ▶+ $

TOXICOLOGY (Consult poison center for specialized dosing)

acetylcysteine (*Mucomyst*): Acetaminophen toxicity: Load 140 mg/kg PO or NG, then 70 mg/kg q4h x 17 doses. May be mixed in water or soda. IV use possible; consult poison center. [Generic/Trade: solution 10%, 20%.] ▶L ♀B ▶? $$$

charcoal (*activated charcoal, Actidose-Aqua, CharcoAid, Charcodate*): 0.5-1.0 g/kg up to 100 g PO. May repeat q4h. [OTC/Generic/Trade: Tabs 250 mg, Caps 260 mg, solution 25 g/ 120 ml.] ▶Not absorbed ♀+ ▶+ $

deferoxamine (*Desferal*): Specialized dosing for acute iron toxicity. ▶K ♀C ▶? $$$$$

dimercaprol (*BAL in oil*): Specialized dosing for arsenic, mercury, gold, lead toxicity. ▶KL ♀C ▶? $$$$$

edetate disodium (*EDTA, Endrate, Meritate*): Lead toxicity. ▶K ♀C ▶- $$$

ethanol: Specialized dosing for methanol, ethylene glycol toxicity. ▶L ♀D ▶+ ?

flumazenil (*Romazicon, Anexate*): benzodiazepine sedation reversal: 0.2 mg IV over 15 sec, then 0.2 mg q1 min prn up to 1 mg total dose. Overdose reversal: 0.2 mg IV over 30 sec, then 0.3-0.5 mg q30 sec prn up to 3 mg total dose. Contraindicated in mixed drug overdose or chronic benzodiazepine use. ▶LK ♀C ▶? $$$

fomepizole (*Antizol*): Ethylene glycol or methanol toxicity. ▶L ♀C ◗? $$$$$

ipecac syrup: Rarely used. Emesis: 30 ml PO for adults, 15 ml if 1-12 yo. [Generic/OTC: syrup.] ▶Gut ♀C ◗? $

methylene blue (*Urolene blue*): Methemoglobinemia: 1-2 mg/kg IV over 5 min. ▶K ♀C ◗? $$

penicillamine (*Cuprimine, Depen*): Specialized dosing for copper toxicity. [Trade: Caps 125, 250 mg; Tabs 250 mg.] ▶K ♀D ◗- $$$

pralidoxime (*Protopam*): Organophosphate toxicity. ▶K ♀C ◗? $$$

sorbitol: Cathartic: 30- 50 ml of 70% sol'n PO. [Generic: oral solution 70%.] ▶Not absorbed ♀+ ◗+ $

succimer (*Chemet*): Lead toxicity in children ≥1 yo: Start 10 mg/kg PO or 350 mg/m^2 q8h x 5 days, then reduce the frequency to q12h x 2 weeks. [Trade: Caps 100 mg.] ▶K ♀C ◗? $$$$$

UROLOGY

Benign Prostatic Hyperplasia

doxazosin (*Cardura*): Start 1 mg PO hs, max 8 mg/day. [Trade: Tabs 1, 2, 4, 8 mg.] ▶L ♀C ◗? $$

finasteride (*Proscar*): 5 mg PO qd [Trade: Tabs 5 mg.] ▶L ♀X ◗- $$$

tamsulosin (*Flomax*): 0.4 mg PO qd, given 30 min after a meal. Maximum 0.8 mg/day. [Trade: Caps 0.4 mg.] ▶LK ♀B ◗- $$

terazosin (*Hytrin*): Start 1 mg PO hs, usual effective dose 10 mg/day, max 20 mg/day. [Generic/Trade: Caps 1, 2, 5, 10 mg.] ▶LK ♀C ◗? $$

Bladder Agents

B&O Supprettes (belladonna and opium): 1 supp PR qd-bid, max 4 doses/day. [Generic/Trade: supp 30 mg [15A], 60 mg [16A].] ▶L ♀C ◗? ©II $$$

flavoxate (*Urispas*): 100-200 mg PO tid/qid. [Trade: Tabs 100 mg.] ▶K ♀B ◗? $$$$

hyoscyamine (*Anaspaz, A-spaz, Cystospaz, ED Spaz, Hyosol, Hyospaz, Levbid, Levsin, Levsinex, Medispaz, Spacol, Spasdel, Symax*): 0.125-0.375 mg PO/SL q4h prn or 0.375-0.75 mg PO q12h (ext release), max 1.5 g/day. [Generic/Trade: Tabs 0.125; sublingual Tabs 0.125 mg; extended release Tabs 0.375 mg; extended release Caps 0.375 mg; elixir 0.125 mg/ 5 ml; drops 0.125 mg/1 ml; Trade only: Tabs 0.15 mg (Hyospaz, Cystospaz).] ▶LK ♀C ◗- $

imipramine (*Tofranil, Tofranil-PM, Impril*): 25-50 mg PO hs. [Generic/Trade: Tabs 10, 25, 50 mg. Trade only: Caps (Tofranil-PM) 75, 100, 125, 150 mg.] ▶L ♀B ◗? $

oxybutynin (*Ditropan, Ditropan XL, Oxybutyn*): 5 mg PO bid/tid or 5-30 mg PO qd (Ext release). [Generic/Trade: Tabs 5 mg; syrup 5 mg/ ml. Trade only: extended release tabs (Ditropan XL) 5, 10, 15 mg.] ▶LK ♀B ◗? $

pentosan polysulfate (*Elmiron*): Interstitial cystitis: 100 mg PO tid. [Trade: Caps 100 mg.] ▶K ♀B ◗? $$$$

phenazopyridine (*Pyridium, Azo-Standard, Urogesic, Prodium, Pyridiate, Urodol, Baridium, UTI Relief, Pyronium, Phenazo Tab*): Dysuria: 200 mg PO tid x 2 days. Turns urine & contact lenses orange. [OTC/Generic/Trade: Tabs 95, 97.2 mg. Generic/Trade: Tabs 100, 200 mg.] ▶K ♀B ◗? $

Prosed/DS (methenamine + phenyl salicylate + methylene blue + benzoic acid + atropine sulfate + hyoscyamine sulfate): 1 tab qid with liberal fluids. [Trade only: Tab 81.6/36.2/10.8/9.0/0.06/0.06 mg] ▶KL ♀C ▶? $$$

Urised (methenamine + phenyl salicylate + atropine + hyoscyamine + benzoic acid + methylene blue): Dysuria: 2 tabs PO qid. Turns urine blue, don't use with sulfa. [Trade: tablet 40.8/18.1/0.03/0.03/4.5/5.4] ▶K ♀C ▶? $$$$

tolterodine (*Detrol*): 1-2 mg PO bid. [Trade: Tabs 1, 2 mg.] ▶L ♀C ▶- $$$

Erectile Dysfunction

alprostadil (*Muse, Caverject, Edex*): 1 intraurethral pellet (Muse) or intracavernosal injection (Caverject, Edex) at lowest dose that will produce erection. [Trade: injection (Edex) 10,20,40 mcg; (Caverject) 6.15,11.9,23.3 mcg. pellet (Muse) 125, 250, 500, 1000 mcg.] ▶L ♀- ▶- $$$$$

sildenafil (*Viagra*): Start 50 mg PO 0.5-4 hours prior to intercourse. Max 1 dose/day. Usual effective range 25-100 mg. Start at 25 mg if >65 years, or liver/renal impairment. Contraindicated with nitrates – fatalities reported. Not FDA approved for women. [Trade: Tabs 25, 50, 100 mg.] ▶LK ♀B ▶- $$$$

Nephrolithiasis

acetohydroxamic acid (*Lithostat*): 250 mg PO tid-qid. [Trade: Tabs 250 mg] ▶K ♀X ▶? $$$

allopurinol (*Zyloprim, Purinol, Alloprin*): 200-300 mg PO qd/bid. [Generic/Trade: Tabs 100, 300 mg.] ▶K ♀C ▶+ $

hydrochlorothiazide (*HCTZ, Esidrix, HydroDIURIL, Oretic, Microzide, Ezide, Hydrocot, Aquazide H*): 50-100 mg PO qd. [Generic/Trade: Tabs 25, 50, 100 mg; solution 50mg/ 5ml. Trade only: Caps 12.5 mg.] ▶L ♀B ▶+ $

potassium citrate (*Polycitra-K, Urocit-K*): Urinary alkalinization: 1 packet in water/juice PO tid/qid. [Trade: Polycitra-K packet K+/citric acid 3300/1002 mg. Polycitra-K oral solution (5 ml = 1100/334 mg). Urocit-K wax Tabs 5, 10 mEq.] ▶K ♀C ▶? $$$

Prostate Cancer

bicalutamide (*Casodex*): 50 mg PO qd. [Trade: Tabs 50 mg.] ▶L ♀X ▶- $$$$$

flutamide (*Eulexin, Euflex*): 250 mg PO q8h. [Trade: Caps 125 mg.] ▶KL ♀D ▶- $$$$$

goserelin (*Zoladex*): 3.6 mg implant SC q28 days, or 10.8 mg SC q12 weeks. [Trade: implants 3.6, 10.8 mg.] ▶L ♀X ▶- $$$$$

leuprolide (*Lupron, Oaklide*): 1 mg SC qd, 7.5 mg IM q month, 22.5 mg IM q3 months, or 30 mg IM q4 months. ▶L ♀X ▶- $$$$$

nilutamide (*Nilandron, Anandron*): 300 mg PO qd for 30 days, then 150 mg qd. [Trade: Tabs 50 mg.] ▶K ♀C ▶? $$$$$

Other Agents

bethanechol (*Urecholine, Duvoid, Myotonachol*): Urinary retention: 10-50 mg PO tid/qid. [Generic/Trade: Tabs 5, 10, 25, 50 mg.] ▶L ♀C ▶? $

desmopressin (*DDAVP, Octostim*): enuresis: 10-40 mcg intranasally hs. Not for children <6 yo. [Trade: Tabs 0.1, 0.2 mg; nasal solution 0.1 mg/ml (10 mcg/ spray).] ▶LK ♀B ▶? $$$$

methylene blue (*Urolene blue*): 65-130 mg PO tid after meals with liberal water. [Trade only: Tabs 65 mg.] ▶Gut/K ♀C ▶? $

t = top of page
m = middle of page
b= bottom of page
D= for brevity in deluxe edition only

15-methyl-pro67b
3TC 19m
5FU 40b,69m
5-HT1 Agonist62t
5-HT3 Antago 52t
6-MP 69m

A

A/T/S 35b
A-200 37m
abacavir 19m
Abbokinase D
Abbreviations 4
abciximab 30t
Abelcet 16m
acarbose 43t
Accolate 78b
Accupril 25b
Accuretic 29m
Accutane 35b
ACE Inhibitor25m
acebutolol 30b
Acel-Imune 58b
Aceon 25b
acetaminophen 10t,13,14,15,62m
acetazolamide 32m,71t
acetic aci50m,50t
acetohy acid 81m
Acetoxyl 35b
acetylcysteine 78b,79b
Acilac 55b
Aciphex 55m
acitretin 37b
Aclovate 39b
Acne Preps 35m
acrivastine D
ActHIB 58b
Acticin 37b
*ActidoseAqua*79b
Actifed Cold 48t
Actigall 57m
Actinex 41t
Actiq 12m
*Activase*34b,63m
activ charcoal79b
Activella 65b
Actonel 41b
Actos 43b
Actron 11m
Acular 71b
acyclovir 18b,38t
Adalat 67m
adapalene 35b
Adderall 76m
Adenocard 26b
adenosine 26b
ADH 57m
Adipex-P 76b
Adriamycin 69m
Adrucil 69m
*Advair Diskus*77b
Advil 11t
AeroBid 78m
Afrin 51m
Agenerase 19b
Aggrastat 30b
*Aggreno*30m,63m
Agoral 55b
Agrylin 30m
AK Tracin 69b
AK-Con 72t
Akineton 62b
AK-Mycin 69b
*AK-Pentolate*71m
AK-Pred 70b
Al hydroxide 10t
Alamast 72t
alatrofloxacin 24t
Albalon 72t
albendazole 18t
Albenza 18t
Albumarc 35t
albumin 35t
Albuminar 35t
albuterol77b,77m
alclometason 39b
Alcomicin 69b
Aldactazide 29m
Aldacton 33t,47m
Aldara 38t
aldesleukin 69m
Aldoclor-250 D
Aldomet 26b
Aldoril D
alendronate 41b
Alertec 76b
Alesse 65
Aleve 11m
Alfenta D
alfentanil D
Alferon N 69m
alitretinoin 40m
Alkeran 69t
Alkylating age69t
Allegra 47m
Allegra-D 48t
Aller-Chlor 47b
Allerdryl 49t,75m,77t
Allerest 72t
Allerfrim 48t
*Allermax Diph*77t
Allermax 75m
Allernix 49t,75m,77t
Alloprin 44t,81m
allopurino44t,81m
Almore 44b
Alocril 72t
Alomide 71b
Alora 64m
alosetron 56m
Alphagan 71t
alprazolam 74b
alprostadil 81t
Alrex 70b
Alromir 77m
Alsoy 45m
Altace 26t
alteplase34b,63m
Alternagel 53t
altretamine 69b
aluminum ace 50t
aluminum OH 53t
Alupent 77m
Alu-tab 53t
Alzheimer's 60m
amantadin20t,63t
Amaryl 42b
Ambien 75b
AmBisome 16m
amcinonide 38,39
Amen 66b
Amerge 62t
Amicar 58t
Amidate 15m
amikacin 16t
Amikin 16t
amiloride 29b,33t
aminocaproic 58t
Aminoglycosid16t
aminolevulini40m
aminophylline D
amiodarone 27t
amitriptyline 72b
amlexanox 50m
amlodipin29b,31b
amobarbital D
amoxapine D
amox clavula 23t
amoxicillin 6,23t,53b
Amoxil 23t
Amphojel 53t
Amphotec 16m
amphotericin 16m,36b
ampicillin 23m
amp sulbacta23m
Ampicin 23m
amprenavir 19b
amyl nitrite D
Anabolic Ster41m
Anafranil 72b
anagrelide 30m
Analgesics 9
*Anandro*69m,81b
Anaprox 11m
Anaspaz 80m
anastrozole 69m
Ancef 20m
Ancobon 16b
Androderm 41m
Androgel 41m
Androgens 41m
Android 41m
Anectine 16t
Anesthesia 15
Anexate 79b
Anexsia 13m
Angio Blocker 26t
anhydr glyce 50m
anistreplase D
Anorexiants 75m
Ansaid 11t
Antabuse 76t
Antacids 53t
Antagon 64b
Anthra-Derm 38t
anthralin 38t
Anthrascalp 38t
Antiadrenergi26m
Anti-Allergy 71b
Anticoagulant57m
Anticonvulsa 60b
Antidepress72,73
Antidiarrheals51b
Anti-Dysrhyth 26b
Antiemetics 52
Antifung 16m,36b
Antihistamines 47
Anti-Hyperli 28,29
Antihypertensi 29
Antimalarials 17t
Antimanic 73b
Antimetabolit69m
Antimicrobials 16
Antimyocoba 17m
Antiparasitics37m
Antiparasitics 18t
Antiplatelet 30t
Antipsoriatics 37b
Antipsychotics 74
antipyrine 49b
Antirheumatics 9t
Antitussives 49m
Antiulcer 53
antivenin-crotal D
antivenin-latrod D
Antivert 63b
Antizol 80t
Anusol 40t
Anzemet 52t
Aparkane 62b
Aphthasol 50m
Aplisol 60m
apraclonidine 71t
Apresazide 29m
Apresoline 29b
Aprodine 48t
APSAC D
Aquachloral 75m
AquaMephyt 46m
Aquatensen D
Aquazide H 81m
ARA-C 69m
Aralen 17t
Aramine D
Arava 9m
ardeparin 57m
Aredia 41b
Arfonad D
Aricept 60m
Arimidex 69m
Aristocort 38,39,42m
Aristospan 42m
Armour Thyroid D
Aromasin 69m
Artane 62b
Arthrotec 10m
artificial tears 72t
*ASA*10m,10t,13b, 14m,14t,30m
Asacol 56b
Asaphen 10m
ascorbic acid 46t
Ascriptin 10t
Asendin D
Asmavent 77m
asparaginase 69b
A-spaz 80m
aspirin 10m,30m, 30m,62m,63m
Astelin 51t
*AsthmaNefrin*79m
Atacand 26t
Atamet 63t
Atapryl 63m
Atarax 49t
Atasol 15t
atenolol 29b,30b
Ativan 61m,75t
atorvastatin 28m
atovaquone 17m
atovaquone 18t
Atromid-S D
atropine 27t,52t, 54b,71m,81t
*Atrovent Nas*51m
Atrovent 79m
attapulgite 51b
aug betame38,39
Augmentin 23t
Auralgan 49b

auranofin 9t
Aurolate 9t
aurothioglucos 9t
Avalide 29m
Avandia 44t
Avapro 26t
Aveeno 41t
Avelox 24t
Aventyl 73t
Avirax 18b
Avlosulfon 17m
Avonex 63b
Axid 53m
Aygestin 67t
Azactam 24b
azatadine 47b,48b
azathioprine 9t
azelaic acid 35b
azelastine 51t
Azelex 35b
azidothymidin 19b
azithromycin 22t
Azmacort 78b
Azopt 71t
Azo-Standard 80b
AZT 19b
aztreonam 24b
Azulfidine 9m,57t

B

B&O Suppret 80m
B12 69t
B6 69t
Bacillus Cal 69m
bacitracin 36m, 36t,69b,70t
baclofen 9m
Bactocill 22b
Bactrim 24t
Bactroban 36m
BAL in oil 79b
balsalazide 56m
banana bag 45m
Banaril 75m,77t
Barbiturates 74,75
Baridium 80b
barium sulfat 35m
basiliximab 60t
Baycol 28m
Bayer 10m,30m
Baygam 58b
BayHep B 58b
BayRab 60t
BayRho-D 60t
Bay Tet 60t
BCG vaccine 58b
BCG 69m
BCNU 69t
B-D Glucose 43t
Beben 42t
becaplermin 40m
Beclodisk 78m
beclomethasone 51t,78m
Beclovent 78m
Beconase 51t
belladonna 80m
Bellergal -S D
Benadryl 49t,50b,75m,77t
benazepril 25m,29b,29m
bendroflumet 29m
Benemid 44m
Benign Prosta 80t
Bensylate 62b,77t
Bentyl 54b
Bentylol 54b
Benuryl 44m
Benylin 49m
Benzac 35b
benzathine p 22m
benzocaine 49b
benzoic acid 81t
benzonatate 49m
benzoyl perox 35b
benztropine m 62b
benztropine 77t
benzylpenicilloy D
bepridil D
beractant D
Beta Agonists 77m
Beta Blockers 30b
Betagan 70b
Betaloc 31m
betamethasone 38,39,42t,68b
Betapace 28t
Betaseron 63b
betaxolol 30b,70b
Betaxon D
bethanechol 81m
Betoptic 70b
Biaxin XL 22t
Biaxin 22t
bicaluta 69m,81b
bicarbonate s 27t
Bicillin CR 22m
Bicillin L-A 22m
BiCNU 69t
Biltricide D
biperiden 62b
bisacodyl 55m
bismuth s 52t,53b
bisoprolol 29b,31t
Bisphosphon 41b
bitolterol 77m
Bladder 80m
Blenoxane 69m
bleomycin 69m
Bleph-10 70t
Blocadren 31m
Bonamine 63b
Bonine 63b
Brethine 67m,77b
Bretylate 27t
bretylium 27t
Bretylol 27t
Brevibloc 31t
Brevicon 65
Brevital 15m
Bricanyl 67m,77b
brimonidine 71t
brinzolamide 71t
Bromaline 48t
Bromatapp 48t
Bromfenex 48t
bromocriptine 46b,63t
brompheniramine 47b,48t
budesonide 51t,78m
bumetanide 32b
Bumex 32b
Buminate 35t
bupivacaine 15b
Buprenex 12t
buprenorphine 12t
bupropio 73m,75b
BuSpar 75m
Buspirex 75m
buspirone 75m
Bustab 75m
busulfan 69t
butabarbital D
butalbital 10t,13b
butenafine 36b
Butisol D
butoconazole 67b
butorphanol 12t

C

C.E.S. 64m
cabergoline 46b
Cafergot 62m
Caffedrine 76m
caffeine 10m,10t, 10b,62m,76m
calamine 40m
Calan 32m
Calcijex 46t
Calcimar 46b
calcipotriene 38t
calcitonin-sal 46b
calcitriol 46t
calcium aceta 44m
calcium carbonat 44m,53t,69t
Calcium blo 31,32
calcium chlor 44m
calcium gluc 44m
calfactant D
Caltine 46b
Camptosar 60m
candesartan 26t
Candistatin 68m
Canestin 68t
capecitabine 69m
Capital wCod 13m
Capoten 25m
Capozide 29m
capsaicin 40m
captopril 25m,29m
Carafate 50b,55t
carbamazepine 60b,73b
carbamide per 50t
Carbapenem 20m
Carbatrol 60b,73b
Carbex 63m
carbidop 63m,63t
carbinoxamine 48
Carbocaine 15b
Carbodec DM 48t
Carbolith 73b
carboplatin 69t
carboprost 67b
Cardene 31b
Cardio-Omeg 29t
Cardiovascular 25
Cardizem 32t
Cardura 26m,80m
carisoprodol 9b,10m,14m
carmustine 69t
carteolol 70b
Cartrol D
carvedilol 31t
casanthranol 56t
cascara 55m
Casodex 69m,81b
castor oil 55m
Cataflam 10b
Catapres TTS 75b,68b
Catapres 26m, 68b,75b,77t
Caverject 81t
CCNU 69t
Ceclor 20b
Cedax 21m
CeeNu 69t
cefaclor 20b
cefadroxil 20m
cefazolin 20m
cefdinir 21t
cefepime 22t
cefixime 21t
Cefizox 21m
Cefobid 21t
cefoperazone 21t
Cefotan 20b
cefotaxime 21t

Index - 83

t = top of page
m = middle of page
b= bottom of page
D= for brevity in deluxe edition only

cefotetan 20b
cefoxitin 20b
cefpodoxime 21t
cefprozil 20b
ceftazidime 21m
ceftibuten 21m
Ceftin 20b
ceftizoxime 21m
ceftriaxone 21m
cefuroxime 20b
Cefzil 20b
Celebrex 10b
celecoxib 10b
Celestone 42t,68b
Celexa 72m
Cellcept 60t
Cenestin 64b
cephalexin 20m
Cephalospo 20-22
Cephulac 55b
Ceptaz 21m
Cerebyx 61t
cerivastatin 28m
Certiva 58b
Cerubidine 69m
Cerumenex 50m
Cervical Ripe 66m
Cervidil 66m
cetirizine 47b
CharcoAid 79b
charcoal 79b
Charcodate 79b
Chemet 80t
Chemstrip 43m
Cheracol D C 48t
Chibroxin 70t
Chlo-Amine 47b
chloral hydra 75m
chlorambucil 69t
chlorampheni 24b
chlordiazepoxide 56b,74b
Chlordrine SR 48t
chlorhexidine 50m
Chloromyceti 24b
chloroquine p 17t
chlorothiazide 33t
chlorpheniramine 47b,48
Chlorproman 74m
chlorpromazi 74m
chlorpropamide D
chlorthalidone 29b,29m,33t

t = top of page
m = middle of page
b= bottom of page
D= for brevity in deluxe edition only

ChlorTrimeto 47b
chlorzoxazone 9b
cholera vacci 58b
cholestyramin 28t
choline 12t
Chronovera 32m
Chronulac 55b
ciclopirox 36b
cidofovir 18b
Cidomycin 16t
cilostazol 58t
Ciloxan 69b
cimetidine 53m
Cipro HC Otic 50t
Cipro 23b
ciprofloxacin 23b,50t,69b
cisapride 56m
cisatracurium 15b
cisplatin 69t
citalopram 72m
Citrucel 55b
cladribine 69m
Claforan 21t
clarithromycin 22t,53b
Claritin 47m
Claritin-D 48t
Clavulin 23t
Clear Eyes 72t
Clearasil 35b
clemastine 47b
Cleocin T 35b
Cleocin 24b,67b
Climara 64m
clindamycin 24b,35b,67b
clinidium 56b
Clinistix 43m
Clinitest 43m
Clinoril 11b
clobetasol 38,39
clocortolone 38,39
Cloderm 38,39
clofazimine D
clofibrate D
Clomid 68b
clomiphene 68b
clomipramine 72b
Clonapam 75t,60b
clonidine 26m, 29m,68b,75b,77t
clopidogrel 30m
clorazepate D
clotrimazole 16m, 36b,38m,50b,68t
cloxacillin D
clozapine 74t
Clozaril 74t
coal tar 40m
codeine 12,13, 14m,48b,48m
Cogentin 62b,77t
Cognex 60b
Colace 55m
Colazal 56m
colchicine 44t
colesevelam 28t
Colestid 28m
colestipol 28m
colfosceril palm D
colistin 50t
CoLytely 56t
Combantrin 18m
CombiPatch 65b
Combipres 29m
Combivent 77b
Combivir 19m
Compazine 52b
Comtan 62b
Comvax 58b
Concerta 76b
Condyline 38m
Condylox 38m
Congest 64m
conj estrogen 66m
Conray 35m
Contac 12-Hr 48t
Contrast Media 35
Copaxone 63b
Cordarone 27t
Cordran 38,39
Coreg 31t
Corgard 31m
Corlopam D
Correctol 55m
Cortaid 38,39
Cortef 42t
Corticaine 38,39
Corticosteroids 38m,38b,42t,70m
cortisone 42t
Cortisporin oti 50t
Cortisporin 38m,70m
Cortizone 38,39
Cortoderm 38,39
Cortone 42t
Cortrosyn 47t
Corvert 27m
Corzide 29m
Cosmegen 69m
Cosopt 71t
cosyntropin 47t
Cotazym 57t
Cotrim 24t
cotrimoxazole 24t
Coumadin 58t
Covera-HS 32m
Cozaar 26m
Creon 57t
Crinone 68m
Crixivan 19b
Crolom 71b
cromolyn 71b,79t
crotamiton 37m
Cuprimine 80t
Curosurf D
Curretab 66b
Cutivate 38,39
cyanocobalam 46t
cyclobenzaprin 9b
Cyclocort 38,39
Cyclogyl 71m
cyclopentolat 71m
cyclophospha 69t
cyclosporine 60t
Cycrin 66b
Cydec Drops 48t
Cylert D
cyproheptadi 47b
Cystografin 35m
Cystospaz 80m
cytarabine 69m
Cytomel 45b
Cytosar-U 69m
Cytotec 54b,66m
Cytovene 18b
Cytoxan 69t

D

d4T 19b
dacarbazine 69t
daclizumab 60t
dactinomycin 69m
Dalacin C 24b
Dalacin T 35b
Dalacin 67b
dalfopristin 25m
Dalgan 12t
Dalmane 74b
dalteparin 57m
danaparoid 57b
danazol 68b
Danocrine 68b
Dantrium D
dantrolene D
dapsone 17m
Daraprim 18m
Darvocet 13b
Darvon 13b,13m
daunorubicin 69m
DaunoXome 69m
Daypro 11b
DDAVP 47t,58m,81m
ddC 19b
ddI 19m
Debrox 50t
Decadron 42t, 63m,68b,79t
Deca-Durabo 41m
Deconamine 48t
Decongestant 49b
Deconsal II 48t
deferoxamine 79b
Delatestryl 41m
delavirdine 19t
Delestrogen 64m
Delsym 49m
Deltasone 42m
Demadex 32b
Demerol 12b
Demser D
Demulen 65
Denavir 38m,50b
denileukin dif 69m
Depacon 61b,73b
Depakene 61b,62m,73b
Depakote 61b,62m,73b
Depen 80t
depGynogen 64m
Depo-Estradi 64m
DepoGen 64m
Depo-Medrol 42m,63b
Deponit 34t
Depo-Provera 66b
Depotest 41m
Depo-Testos 41m
Deproic 61b,62m,73b
Dermatology 35
Dermatop 38,39
Dermazin 36m
Dermolate 38,39
Dermovate 38,39
deserpidine D
Desferal 79b
desipramine 72b
desmopressin 47t,58m,81m
Desocort 38,39
Desogen 65
desogestrel 65
desonide 38,39
DesOwen 38,39
desoximeta 38,39
Desquam 35b
Desyrel 73m
Detrol 81t
Detussin 48t
dexamethasone 42t,63m,68b, 70b,79t
Dexason 42t,63m
dexchlorpheni 47b
Dexedrine 76b
DexFerrum 44b
Dexiron 44b
Dexone 42t
dextran 35t
dextroamphetamine 76b,76m
dextrometh 48,49
dextrose 43t
Dextrostat 76b
Dextrostix 43m
dezocine 12t
DHE 45 62m
DHPG 18b
DHT 46t
DiaBeta 43t
Diabinese D
Diamox 32m,71t
Diascan 43m
Diasorb 51b
Diastat 9b,60b
Diastix 43m
diatrizoate 35m
diazepam 9b,60b,75t
diazoxide 43m
Dibenzyline D
dibucaine 40t
dichloralphen 62m
diclofenac 10b,10m,71b
dicloxacillin 22b
dicyclomine 54b
didanosine 19m
Didronel 41b
difenoxin D
Differin 35b
diflorasone 38,39
Diflucan 16m,69t
diflunisal 10b
Digibind 27m
Digitek 27t
digoxin 27t
digoxin Fab 27m
dihydroergot 62m
dihydrotachys 46t
diiodohydroxyq D
Dilacor 32t
Dilantin 61m
Dilatrate-SR 33m
Dilaudid 12m
Dilia XT 32t
diltiazem 32t
Dimaphen 48t
dimenhydrinate 49t,52m
dimercaprol 79b
Dimetapp Alle 47b
Dimetapp 48t

t = top of page
m = middle of page
b= bottom of page
D= for brevity in deluxe edition only

dinoprostone 60m
Diocarpine 71m
Diodoquin D
Diovan HCT 29m
Diovan 26m
Dipentum 57t
Diphen 61m,75m
diphenhydramine 49t,75m,77t
diphenoxylate 62t
diphtheria 58b
diphtheria-tet 58b
dipivefrin 71t
Diprivan 15m
Diprolene 38,39
Diprosone 38,39
dipyridamole 30m,63m
dirithromycin D
Disalcid 11b
disopyramide D
disulfiram 76t
Ditropan 80b
Diucardin D
Diuretics 32
Diuril 33t
Diutensen-R D
Dixarit 75b,77t
dobutamine 34t
Dobutrex 34t
docetaxel 69m
docusate 55m,56t
dofetilide 27m
dolasetron 52t
Dolobid 10b
Dolophine 12b,76t
DomeboroOtic 50t
donepezil 60m
Donnagel 51b
Donnatal 54b
Donnazyme 57t
dopamine 34m
Dopaminergic 63t
dornase alfa 79t
Doryx 17m,24m,35b
dorzolamide 71t
Dostinex 46b
Dovonex 38t
doxazos 26m,80m
doxepin 40m,73t
doxercalciferol 46t
Doxia 69m
Doxil 69m
doxorubicin 69m
Doxycin 17m,24m
doxycycline 17m,24m,35b
doxylamine 52m
Dramamine 49t,52m
Dristan 12Hr 51m
Drithocreme 30t
dronabinol 52b
droperidol 52b
Drug Depend 75b
Drugs in preg 66t
DTaP 58b,58m
DTIC-Dome 69t
Dulcolax 55m
Duradrin 62m
Duragesic 12m
Duralith 73b
Duranest 15b
Duratex 48t
Duratuss 48t
Duricef 20m
Duvoid 81m
Dyazide 29m
Dynabac D
Dynacin 24b
DynaCirc CR 31b
DynaCirc 31b
Dynapen 22b
Dyrenium D
Dytuss 75m,77t

E

E Pam 60b,75t
Ear Preps 49b
echothiophat 71m
EC-Naprosyn 11m
econazole 36b
Ecotrin 10m,30m
ED Spaz 80m
Edecrin 32b
edetate disodi 79b
Edex 81t
edrophonium 63b
EDTA 79b
EES 22m
efavirenz 19t
Effexor XR 73t
Effexor 73t
Efidac/24 49b
Efudex 40b
Elavil 72b
Eldepryl 63m
Eldopaque 40b
Eldoquin 40b
Elimite 37b
Elixophyllin 78b
Ellence 69m
Elmiron 80b
Elocon 38,39
Elspar 69b
Eltroxin 45b
Emcyt 69m
Emetrol 52b
Eminase D
EMLA 40b
Empirin wCod 13b
Empirin 10m,30m
E-mycin 22m
enalapril 25b,29b,29m
Enbrel 9t
Endantadine 63t
Endocodone 13t
Endocrine/Met 41
Endrate 79b
Enduron D
Enduronyl Forte D
Enduronyl D
Enfamil 45m
Engerix-B 58b
Enlon 63b
enoxacin 23b
enoxaparin 57b
ENT Combos 48
ENT 47
entacapone 62b
Entex LA 48m
Entex PSE 48m
Entex 48m
Entozyme 57t
Entrophen 30m
ephedrine 34m
Epiject 61b,62m,73b
epinephrine racemic 79m
epinephrine 27m,34m,79t
epirubicin 69m
Epitol 60b,73b
Epival 61b,62m,73b
Epivir 19m
Epivir-HBV 19m
epoetin alfa 58m
Epogen 58m
epoprostenol D
Eprex 58m
eprosartan 26t
eptifibatide 30m
Equalactin 56t
Ercaf 62m
Erectile dysfu 81t
Ergamisol 69b
ergotamine 62m
Eryc 22m
Erycette 35b
Eryderm 35b
Erygel 35b
Erythrocin 22m
erythromycins 22m,35b,69b
erythropoietin 58m
Esclim 64m
Esgic 10t
Esidrix 33t,81m
Eskalith 73b
esmolol 31t
Esoterica 40b
estazolam 75t
esterified estrogens 64t,65b
Estinyl 64b
Estrace 64m,68t
Estraderm 64m
estradiol 64m,65b,66m,68t
EstraGyn 5 64b
Estra-L 40 64m
estramustine 69m
Estratab 64t
Estratest 65b
Estring 68t
estrogen crea 68t
estrogens 64
estrone 64b
estropipate 64b
Estrostep Fe 65
etanercept 9t
ethacrynic aci 32b
ethambutol 17b
ethanol 79b
ethinyl estr 64b,65
ethionamide 17b
Ethmozine D
ethosuximide 61t
ethynodiol 65
Etibi 17b
etidocaine 15b
etidronate 41b
etodolac 10b
etomidate 15m
etoposide 69m
Etrafon D
Euflex 81b
Euglucon 43t
Eulexin 69m,81b
Eurax 37m
Everone 41m
Evista 47t,67t
Excedrin Mig 62m
Exelon 60b
exemestane 69m
Exgest LA 48m
Exosurf Neonat D
Expectorants 49m
Exsel 41t
Ezide 81m

F

factor VIII,IX 58m
famciclovir 19t
famotidine 53m
Famvir 19t
Fareston 69m
fat emulsion 45m
Feen-a-Mint 55m
felbamate 61t
Felbatol 61t
Feldene 11b
felodipin 29m,31b
Femara 69m
Femcare 68t
FemHRT 1/5 65b
Femizol 68m
FemPatch 64m
Femstat 3 67b
Fenesin DM 48m
fenofibrate 28b
fenoldopam D
fenoprofen D
fentanyl 12m,15m
FeoSol 44b
Fergon 44m
Fer-in-Sol 44b
Ferrlecit 45m
ferrous fumara 65
ferrous gluco 44m
ferrous polysa 44b
ferrous sulfate 44b
Fexicam 11b
fexofenadine 47m,48t
Fiberall 56t
FiberCon 56t
filgrastim 58m
finasteride 40b,80m
Fioricet wCod 13b
Fioricet 10t
Fiorinal wCod 13b
Fiorinal 10t
FK 506 60m
Flagyl 18m,25t
Flarex 70b
flavoxate 80m
flecainide D
Fleet enema 56m
Fleet Castor 55m
Fleet Mineral 55b
Fleet Phosph 56m
Flexeril 9b
Flolan D
Flomax 80m
Flonase 51m
Florinef 42t
Flovent 78m
Floxin Otic 50t
Floxin 23b
floxuridine 69m
fluconazole 16m,69t

86 - Index

t = top of page
m = middle of page
b= bottom of page
D= for brevity in deluxe edition only

flucytosine 16b
Fludara 69m
fludarabine 69m
fludrocortison 42t
Flumadine 20m
flumazenil 79b
flunisolide 51m,78m
fluocinolone38,39
Fluoderm 38,39
Fluogen 59t
fluoride 44b
fluorometholo70b
Fluoroplex 40b
fluoroura40b,69m
fluoxetine72m,77t
fluoxymester41m
fluphenazine74m
flurandrenol38,39
flurazepam 74b
flurbiprofen 11t
FluShield 59t
flutamide69m,81b
fluticasone 38,39, 51m,77b,78m
fluvastatin 28m
Fluviral 59t
Fluvirin 59t
fluvoxamine 72m
Fluzone 59t
FML Forte 70b
FML 70b
folate 46t
folic acid 46t,69t
Folvite 46t
fomepizole 80t
fomivirsen D
formulas,ped45m
Formulas 7,8
Fortaz 21m
Fortovase 20t
Fosamax 41b
foscarnet 18b
Foscavir 18b
fosfomycin 24b
fosinopril 25b
fosphenytoin 61t
Fragmin 57m
Froben 11t
FSH/LH 69t
FUDR 69m
Fulvicin-U/F 16b
Fungizone 16m,36b
Furadantin 25t
furazolidone D
furosemide 32b
Furoxone D

G

gabapentin 61t
Gabitril 61b
gadodiamide 35m
gadopentetat35m
Gamimune 58b
Gammagard 58b
Gammar 58b
Gamulin Rh 69t
ganciclovir 18b
ganirelix acet 64b
Gani-Tuss 48m
Gantanol 24m
Gantrisin Pediatric 24m
Garamycin 16t,36t,69b
Gastrocrom 79t
Gastroenterolo51
Gastrografin 35m
Gas-X 55t
gatifloxacin 24t
*Gaviscon Pre*53m
G-CSF 58m
gemcitabine 69m
gemfibrozil 29t
Gemzar 69m
Genora 1/35 65
Genora 1/50 65
Genotropin 47t
gentamicin 16t,36t,69b
Gent-L-Tip 56m
Gentran 35t
Gen-Xene D
GI cocktail 54b
glatiramer 63b
Glaucoma 70,71
Gliadel 69t
glimepiride 42b
glipizide 42b
Glitazone 43b,44t
GlucaGen 43m
glucagon 43m
Glucometer 43m
Gluconorm 44t
Glucophage 43b
glucose test 43m
Glucostix 43m
Glucotrol XL 42b
Glucotrol 42b
Glucovance 43m
Glutose 43t
glyburide43m,43t
glycerin 55b
Glycon 43b
Glynase Pres 43t
Glyset 43b
GM-CSF 58m
GnRH Agonis64b
gold sodium thi 9t
GoLytely 56t
gonadotropins69t
goserelin 64b,69m,81b
Gout-Related 44t
gramicidin 70t
granisetron 52m
Gravol 49t
green goddes54b
Grifulvin-V 16b
griseofulvin 16b
growth hormo 47t
guaifenesin 48
Guaifenex 48m
Guaitex 48m
guanabenz D
guanadrel D
guanethidine D
guanfacine 77t
Guiatus 48m,49m
Guiatussin 48m
Gynazole-1 67b
Gynecure 68b
*Gyne-Lotrimin*68t
Gynogen 64m

H

H2 Antagoni 53m
Habitrol 76m
haemophilus 58b
halcinonide 38,39
Halcion 75m
Haldol 74m
Halfprin 30m
halobetasol 38,39
Halog 38,39
haloperidol 74m
haloprogin 36b
Halotestin 41m
Halotex 36b
Halotussin 48m
Havrix 58b
H-BIG 58b
HCTZ 29b, 29m,33t,81m
Hecterol 46t
Helicobacter pylori 53,54
Helidac 53b
Hemabate 67b
Hematology 57
Hemorrhoid 40t
Hepalean 57b
heparin 57b
hepatitis A va58b
hepatitis B im58b
hepatitis B va58b
Heptovir 19m
Herceptin 69m
Hespan 35t
hetastarch 35t
Hexabrix 35m
Hexadrol 42t,63m
Hexalen 69b
Hextend 35t
HibTITER 58b
Hiprex D
Histinex HC 48m
Histussin D 48m
*Histussin HC*48m
Hivid 19b
homatropine 49m,71m
Hormone repl65b
Hormones 69m
Humalog 43m
human 60t
Humatrope 47t
Humegon 69t
Humibid DM 48m
Humibid LA 49m
Humulin 43m
*Hybolin Deca*41m
Hycamtin 69m
Hycodan 49m
Hycort 38,39
hydralazine 29b,29m
Hydrea 69m
hydrochlorothiazide 33t,81m
Hydrocil 56t
hydrocodone 13,14,48,49
hydrocortisone 38,39,40t,42t, 50m,50t,70m
Hydrocot 81m
HydroDIURIL 33t,81m
hydroflumethiazD
hydromorpho12m
hydroquinone40b
hydroxychloroq 9t
hydroxyproge66b
hydroxyurea 69m
hydroxyzine 49t
Hygroton 33t
Hylorel D
Hylutin 66b
hyoscyamine 54b,80m,81t
Hyosol 80m
Hyospaz 80m
Hypaque 35m
Hyperstat D
Hypotears 72t
HypRho-D 69t
Hytrin 26b,80m
Hytuss 49m
Hyzaar 29m

I

ibuprofen 11t,14b
ibutilide 27m
Idamycin 69m
idarubicin 69m
Ifex 69t
ifosfamide 69t
Ilotycin 69b
Imdur 33b
imipenem-cil 20m
imipramin 73t,80b
imiquimod 38t
Imitrex 62t
immune globu58b
Immunization 58b
Immunoglobu59b
Immunology 58
Immunomod 69m
Immunosuppr 60t
Imodium AD 52t
Imodium 52t
Imogam 60t
Imovax 58m
Impril 73t,80b
Imuran 9t
inamrinone D
Inapsine 52b
indapamide 33m
Inderal 31m
Inderide LA 29m
Inderide 29m
indinavir 19b
Indocid 11t,67m
Indocin IV D
Indocin SR 11t
Indocin 11t,67m
indomethacin 11t,67m
Indotec 11t
Infanrix 58b
Infasurf D
InFed 44b
Infergen D
*Inflamase For*70b
infliximab 56m
influenza vacc59t
Infufer 44b
INH 17b
Inhaled Stero78m
Innohep 57b
Inocor D
Inotropes 34t
Insta-Glucose 43t
insulin 43m
Intal 79t
Integrilin 30m

t = top of page
m = middle of page
b= bottom of page
D= for brevity in deluxe edition only

interferon alf 60m
interferon bet 63b
Interleukin-2 69m
Intralipid 45m
Intron A 69m
Intropin 34m
Inversine D
Invirase 20t
iodine D
iodoquinol D
iohexol 35m
Ionamin 76b
iopamidol 35m
Iopidine 71t
iothalamate 35m
ioversol 35m
ioxaglate 35m
ipecac syrup 80t
ipratropium n51m
ipratropium 77b,79m
irbesarta 26t,29m
irinotecan 69m
iron dextran 44b
Ismelin D
ISMO 33b
isocarboxazid D
isoetharine D
isomethepte 62m
Isomil 45m
isoniazid 17b,18t
isoproterenol 27m
Isoptin 32m
Isopto Atropi 71m
Isopto Carpi 71m
Isopto Cetam 70t
Isopto Homat 71m
Isordil 33m
isosorbide 33m
Isotamine 17b
isotretinoin 35b
Isovue 35m
isoxsuprine D
isradipine 31b
Isuprel 27m
itraconazole 16b
ivermectin 18t

J

Japanese enc 59t
JE-Vax 59t

K

Kabikinase 34b
Kadian 12b
Kaopectate 51b
Kayexalate 47t
Keflex 20m
Keftab 20m
Kefurox 20b
Kefzol 20m
Kenalog 38,39, 42m,50b
Keppra 61m
Kerlone 30b
Kestrone 5 64b
Ketalar 15m
ketamine 15m
ketoconazole 17t,37t
ketoprofen 11m
ketorolac 11m,71b
ketotifen 71b
Klaron 35b
Klean-Prep 56t
Klonopin 60b,75t
Kondremul 55b
K-Phos 45t
Ku-Zyme 57t
Kwellada-P 37b
Kytril 52m

L

labetalol 31t
Lac-Hydrin 40b
Lacrilube 72t
Lactaid 56b
lactase enzy 56b
lactic acid 40b
lactulose 55b
Lamictal CD 61t
Lamictal 61t
Lamisil 17t,37m
lamivudine 19m
lamotrigine 61t
Lamprene D
Lanoxicaps 27t
Lanoxin 27t
lansoprazole 53b,55t
Lantus 43m
Laradopa 63t
Lariam 17m
Lasix 32b
latanoprost 71m
Laxatives 55m
Ledercillin VK 22b
leflunomide 9m
lepirudin 58t
Lescol 28m
letrozole 69m
Leukeran 69t
Leukine 58m
Leukotriene 78b
leuprolide 64b,69m,81b
Leupron 69m
Leustatin 69m
levalbuterol 77m
levamisole 69b
Levaquin 23b
Levate 72b
Levatol D
Levbid 80m
levetiracetam 61m
Levlen 65
Levlite 65
levobetaxolol D
levobunolol 70b
levocabastine 71b
levodopa 63m,63t,63t
LevoDromora 12b
levofloxacin 23b
levonorgestrel 65
Levophed 34m
Levora 65
levorphanol 12b
Levo-T 45b
Levotec 45b
Levothroid 45b
levothyroxine 45b
Levoxyl 45b
Levsin 54b,80m
Levsinex 80m
Levulan Kera 40m
Lexxel 29m
Librax 56b
Librium 74b
Lidex 38,39
Lidex-E 38,39
lidocaine visc 50b
lidocaine 15b,27m,40b
Lidoderm 40b
Limbitrol D
lindane 37m
linezolid 25t
Lioresal 9m
liothyronine 45b
liotrix 45b
Lipitor 28m
Liposyn 45m
lisinopril 25b,29b
Lithane 73b
lithium 73b
Lithobid 73b
Lithonate 73b
Lithostat 81m
Livostin 71b
Lo/Ovral 65
Local Anesthe 15b
LoCHOLEST 28t
Locoid 38,39
Lodine 10b
lodoxamide 71b
Loestrin 65
lomefloxacin 23b
Lomotil 52t
lomustine 69t
Loniten 30t
Loperacap 52t
loperamide 52t
Lopid 29t
LopressHCT 29m
Lopressor 31m
Loprox 36b
Lorabid 21t
loracarbef 21t
loratadine 47m,48t
lorazepa 61m,75t
Lorcet 13b
Lortab 14t
losartan 26m,29m
Losec 55t
Lotemax 70b
LotensinHCT 29m
Lotensin 25m
loteprednol 70b
Lotrel 29b
Lotrimin 36b
Lotrisone 38m
Lotronex 56m
lovastatin 28m
Lovenox 57b
Low-molecul 57m
Low-Ogestrel 65
Loxapac 74m
loxapine 74m
Loxitane 74m
Lozol 33m
L-thyroxine 45b
Ludiomil D
Lugol's Solution D
Luminal 61m
Lupron 64b,81b
Luride 44b
Lustra 40b
Luvox 72m
Lyderm 38,39
lyme vaccine 59t
LYMErix 59t
Lysodren 69b
Lyteprep 56t

M

Maalox 53m
Macrobid 25t
Macrodantin 25t
Macrodex 35t
Macrolides 22t
mafenide 36t
Mag-200 45t
magaldrate 53m
Maganate 44b
magic mouth 50b
magne citrate 55b
magne gluco 44b
magne hydro 55b
magnes oxide 45t
magne salicyl 12t
magnesium sulfate 45t,67m
Magnevist 35m
Mag-Ox 400 45t
Magtrate 44b
Malarone 17m
malathion 37b
Mandelamine D
mannitol 63b
Mantoux 60m
maprotiline D
Marcaine 15b
Marine Lipid C 29t
Marinol 52b
Marmine 52m
Marplan D
masoprocol 41t
Matulane 69t
Mavik 26t
Max EPA 45m
Maxair 77b
Maxalt MLT 62t
Maxalt 62t
Maxaquin 23b
Maxeran 52b
Maxiflor 38,39
Maxipime 22t
Maxitrol 70b
Maxivate 38,39
Maxzide 29b
Maxzide-25 29b
Mazepin 60b,73b
MD-Gastrovi 35m
measles 59t
Mebaral D
mebendazole 18m
mecamylamine D
mechloretham 69t
Meclicot 63b
meclizine 63b
meclofenama 11m
Medispaz 80m
Medivert 63b
Medrol 42m,63b
medroxyprogesterone 66b,66m
mefloquine 17m
Mefoxin 20b
Megace 66b
megestrol 66b
Melanex 40b
Mellaril 74b
meloxicam 11m
melphalan 69t
Menest 64t
Meni-D 63b

t = top of page
m = middle of page
b= bottom of page
D= for brevity in deluxe edition only

meningococca59t
Menogen 65b
Menomune 59t
Mentax 36b
meperidine 12b
mephentermine D
mephobarbital D
Mephyton 46m
mepivacaine 15b
Mepron 18t
mequinol 41t
mercaptopuri69m
Meridia 57t,77t
Meritate 79b
meropenem 20m
Merrem IV 20m
mesalamine 56b
Mesasal 56b
mesoridazine D
Mestinon 64t
mestranol 65
Metadate ER 76b
Metamucil 56t
Metandren 41m
Metaprel 77m
metaproteren77m
metaraminol D
Metastron 69b
metaxalone 9b
metform 43b,43m
methacholine D
methadon12b,76t
*Methados*12b,76t
methenamine 81t
Methergine 67b
methimazole 45b
Methitest 41m
methocarbamol 9b,10m
methohexital 15m
methotre 9m,69m
methoxamine D
methyclothiazid D
methylcellulo 55b
methyldopa 26b
methylene blue 80t,81m,81t
methylergono67b
Methylin 76b
methylphenid 76b
methylpredniso-lone 42m,63b
ethyltestoster-one 41m,65b
methysergide D
Meticorten 42m
metocloprami 52b
metolazone 33m
metoprolol 29m,31m
Metreton 42m
MetroGel 36m
*MetroGelVag*68m
metronidazole 18m,25t,36m, 53b,68m
metyrosine D
Mevacor 28m
mexiletine D
Mexitil D
Mezlin 23m
mezlocillin 23m
Miacalcin 46b
Micardis 26m
Micatin 37t
miconazo37t,68m
Micozole 68m
MICRhoGAM 60t,69t
Micronase 43t
MicroNefrin 79m
Micronor 65
*Microzide*33t,81m
Midamor 33t
midazola 15m,75t
midodrine 34m
Midrin 62m
miglitol 43b
Migraine Rx 62t
Migranal 62m
Milk of Magn 55b
milrinone 34m
mineral oil40t,55b
Minerals 44m
Mini-Gamulin 69t
Minipress 26b
Minitran 34t
Minizide 29b
Minocin 24b
minocycline 24b
Minox 41t
minoxidil 30t,41t
Mintezol D
Miralax 56t
Mirapex 63t
Mircette 65
mirtazapine 73m
misoprostol 10m,54b,66m
Mithracin 69m
mithramycin 69m
mitomycin 69m
mitotane 69b
Mitotic Inhibit69m
mitoxantrone69m
Mivacron 15b
mivacurium 15b
M-M-R II 59t
Moban 74m
Mobic 11m
modafinil 76b
Modecate 74m
Modicon 65
Moditen 74m
Moduret 29b
Moduretic 29b
moexipril 25b,29b
molindone 74m
mometason38,39
mometasone51m
Monazole 68m
*Monistat*68m,68b
MonistatDerm 37t
Monitan 30b
Monoket 33b
Monopril 25b
montelukast 78b
Monurol 24b
moricizine D
morphine sulf12b
Motofen D
Motrin 11t
Mouth & Lip 50m
moxifloxacin 24t
MS Contin 12b
MSIR 12b
*Mucomys*78b,79b
Mucosil 78b
multivitamins46m
mumps & rube59t
mupirocin 36m
Murine Ear 50t
Muscle Relax 9m
Muse 81t
Mustargen 69t
Mutamycin 69m
MVI 46m
Myambutol 17b
Mycelex 16m, 36b,50b,68t
Mycifradin 56b
Mycobutin 17b
Mycolog II 38m
mycophenola 60t
Mycostatin 17t, 37t,50b,68m
Mydfrin 71b
Mydriacyl 71b
Mydriatics/Cy71m
Mykrox 33m
Mylanta 53t,53m
Myleran 69t
Mylicon 55t
*Myotonachol*81m
Mysoline 61m
*Mytussin DM*48m
M-Zole 68m
NABI-HB 58b

N

nabumetone 11m
nadolol 29m,31m
Nadostine 17t
nafarelin 65m
nafcillin 22b
naftifine 37t
Naftin 37t
nalbuphine 12t
Nalcrom 79t
Naldecon 48m
Naldelate 48m
*Nalfon Pulvules*D
nalidixic acid 23b
Nallpen 22b
nalmefene 14b
naloxone 15t
naltrexone 76t
nandrolone d41m
naphazoline 72t
Naphcon 72t
Naprelan 11m
Naprosyn 11m
naproxen 11m
Naqua D
naratriptan 62t
Narcan 15t
Nardil D
Nasacort 51b
Nasal Preps 51t
NaSal 51b
Nasalide 51m
Nasarel 51m
Nasonex 51m
Naturetin D
Navane D
Navelbine 69b
Naxen 11m
Nebcin 16t
NebuPent 18m
Necon 65
nedocro 72t,79m
nefazodone 73m
NegGram 23b
nelfinavir 20t
Nelova 65
Nembutal 75m
neomycin 36m, 38m,50m,50t, 56b,70b,70m,70t
Neoral 60t
Neosar 69t
*Neospori*36m,70t
neostigmine 64t
Neo-Synephrine 34m,51m,71b
Nephrolithias81m
Nephron 79m
Neumega 58m
Neupogen 58m
Neurology 60
Neurontin 61t
Neutra-Phos 45t
nevirapine 19m
niacin 29t,46m
Niacor 29t
Niaspan 29t
nicardipine 31b
Nicoderm 76m
Nicolar 29t
Nicorette DS 76t
Nicorette 76t
nicotine 76t,76m
nicotinic acid 29t
*Nicotrol Inhale*76t
Nicotrol NS 76m
Nicotrol 76m
NidaGel 36m
nifedipin 31b,67m
Niferex 44b
*Nilandro*69m,81b
Nilstat 17t
nilutamid69m,81b
Nimbex 15b
nimodipine 64t
Nimotop 64t
Nipent 69m
Nipride 30t
nisoldipine 32t
Nitrates 33m
NitroBid IV 33b
Nitro-bid 33b
Nitrodisc 34t
Nitro-Dur 34t
nitrofurantoin 25t
nitroglyce 33b,34t
Nitroglyn 34t
Nitroguard D
Nitrol 33b
Nitrolingual 33b
Nitrong 34t
Nitropress 30t
nitroprusside 30t
NitroQuick 33b
Nitrostat 33b
Nix 37b
nizatadine 53m
Nizoral 17t,37t
NoDoz 76m
Nolvadex 47m,67t,69m
Nonsteroidal 10m
Norco 14t
Norcuron 16t
Nordette 65
Norditropin 47t
norepinephri 34m
norethindro65,67t
Norflex 9b

t = top of page
m = middle of page
b= bottom of page
D= for brevity in deluxe edition only

norfloxaci 23b,70t
Norgesic 10m
norgestim 65,66m
norgestrel 65
Norinyl 65
Noritate 36m
Norlutate 67t
Normiflo 57m
Normodyne 31t
Noroxin 23b,70t
Norpace D
Norplant D
Norpramin 72b
Nor-Q.D. 65
nortriptyline 73t
Norvasc 31b
Norventyl 73t
Norvir 20t
Nostril 51m
Nostrilla 51m
Nova Rectal 75m
Novafed A 48m
Novantrone 69m
Novolin 43m
Novolog 43m
Novoxapam 75t
Nubain 12t
Numby Stuff 40b
Numorphan 13m
Nupercainal 40t
Nuprin 11t
Nursoy 45m
Nutritionals 45m
Nutropin 47t
Nyaderm 17t
nystatin 17t,37t, 38m,50b,68m

O

Oaklide 81b
oatmeal 41t
OB/GYN 64
OBY-Trim 76b
Ocean 51b
Octostim 47t,81m
octreotide 66b
Ocuflox 70t
Ocular Deco 71b
Ocupress 70b
ofloxacin 23b,50t,70t
Ogen 64b,68t
Ogestrel 65
olanzapine 74t
olopatadine 72t
olsalazine 57t
omega-3 29t,45m
omeprazole 55t
Omnicef 21t
OmniHIB 58b
Omnipaque 35m
Omniscan 35m
Oncaspar 69b
Oncology 69
Oncovin 69b
ondansetron 52m
Ontak 69m
Ophthaine 72t
Ophthalmology 69
Ophthetic 72t
Opioids 10-13
opium tincture D
opium 80m
oprelvekin 58m
Opticrom 71b
Optimine 47b
Optiray 35m
Orafen 11m
Oral contracep 65
Oralet 15m
OramorphSR 12b
Orap D
Orbenin D
Oretic 33t,81m
Orgaran 57b
Orimune 99t
Orinase D
orlistat 57t
Ornade 48m
orphenadrine 9b,10m
Ortho Dienest 68t
Ortho Tri-Cycl 65
Ortho Cept 65
Ortho-Cyclen 65
Ortho-Est 64b
Ortho-Novum 65
Ortho-Prefest 66m
Orudis 11m
Oruvail 11m
Os-Cal 44m
oseltamivir 20t
Osmitrol 63b
Otobiotic 50t
Ovcon-35 65
Ovide 37b
Ovral 65
Ovrette 65
oxacillin 22b
oxaprozin 11b
oxazepam 75t
oxcarbazepin 61m
oxiconazole 37t
Oxistat 37t
Oxizole 37t
Oxpam 75t
Oxybutyn 80b
oxybutynin 80b
oxycodone 13t,14m,14t
OxyContin 13t
OxyFAST 13t
OxyIR 13t
oxymetazolin 51m
oxymorphon 13m
oxytocin 66m,67b

P

Pacerone 27t
paclitaxel 69m
palivizumab D
Pamelor 73t
pamidronate 41b
Panadol 15t
Pancrease 57t
pancreatin 57t
pancrelipase 57t
pancuronium 15b
Pandel 38,39
Panretin 40m
Pantoloc 55m
pantoprazole 55m
papaverine D
Paraflex 9b
Parafon Forte 9b
Paraplatin 69t
paregoric D
paricalcitol 46m
Parkinsons 62,63
Parlodel 46b,63t
Parnate D
paroxetine 72b
Parvolex 78b
Patanol 72t
Pavulon 15b
Paxil 72b
PediaCare Inf 49b
Pediapred 42m
Pediazole 22m,24m
Pediotic 50m
Peds drugs 6,7
PedvaxHIB 58b
pegaspargase 69b
pemirolast 72t
pemoline D
penbutolol D
penciclovir 38m,50b
Penetrex 23b
penicillamine 80t
penicillin G 22b
penicillin V 22b
Penicillins 22,23
Penlac 36b
Pentacarinat 18m
Pentam 18m
pentamidine 18m
Pentasa 56b
pentazocine 12t,14m
pentobarbital 75m
Pentolair 71m
pentosan pol 80b
pentostatin 69m
Pentothal 15m
pentoxifylline 58m
Pen-Vee K 22b
Pepcid AC 53m
Pepcid 53m
Peptic Relief 53b
Pepto-Bismol 52t
Peptol 53m
Percocet 14t
Percodan 14t
Percolone 13t
pergolide 63t
Pergonal 69t
Periactin 47b
Peri-Colace 56t
Peridex 50m
Peridol 74m
perindopril 25b
Periogard 50m
Periostat 17m,24m
Permax 63t
permethrin 37b
Permitil 74m
perphenazine D
Persantine 30m
PGE1 66m
PGE2 66m
Phazyme 55t
Phenazo Tab 80b
phenazopyridi 80b
phenelzine D
Phenergan 48m,49t,52b
pheniramine 72t
phenobarbital 54b,61m
phenoxybenza D
Phentercot 76b
phentermine 76b
phentolamine 30t
Phentride 76b
phenyl salicyl 81t
phenylephrine 34m,48b,48m, 48t,51m,71b
phenylpropanol-amine 48b, 48m,48t,49b
phenyltoloxamin 48b,48m
phenytoin 61m
PhosLo 44m
Phospholine 71m
phosphorated 52b
phosphorous 45t
Photofrin 69b
phytonadione 46m
Pilocar 71m
pilocarpine 71m
Pilopine HS 71m
pimozide D
pindolol 31m
Pinworm 18m
Pin-X 18m
pioglitazone 43b
piperac tazo 23m
piperacillin 23m
piperonyl butox-ide 37b,37m
Pipracil 23m
pirbuterol 77b
piroxicam 11b
Pitocin 66m,67b
Pitressi 47m,57m
plague vaccin 59t
Plaquenil 9t
plasma protein 35t
Plasmanate 35t
Plasmatein 35t
Platinol 69t
Plavix 30m
Plendil 31b
Pletal 58t
plicamycin 69m
Pneumo 23 59t
pneumococc v 59t
Pneumovax 59t
Pnu-Imune 59t
Podocon-25 38m
Podofilm 38m
podofilox 38m
Podofin 38m
podophyllin 38m
Polaramine 47b
poliovirus vac 59t
polycarbophil 56t
Polycitra-K 81m
polyethylene g 56t
Polygam 58b
Polyhistine D
Polymox 23t
polymyxin 36m, 50m,50t,70b, 70m,70t
Polyspori 36m,70t
Polytar 40m
polythiazide 29b
Polytrim 70t
Pontocaine 72t
porfimer 69b
potassium 45m
PPD 60m
pralidoxime 80t

t = top of page
m = middle of page
b= bottom of page
D= for brevity in deluxe edition only

pramipexole 63t
pramoxine 40t
Prandase 43t
Prandin 44t
Pravachol 28m
pravastatin 28m
praziquantel D
prazosin 26b,29b
Precose 43t
Pred Forte 70b
Pred Mild 70b
prednicarb 38,39
prednisolone 42m,70b
prednisone 42m
Pred-Pak 42m
Prelone 42m
Premarin 64m,68t
Premesis-Rx 69t
Premphase 66m
Prempro 66m
Pre-Pen D
Prepidil 66m
Pressors 34t
Pretz 51b
Prevacid 55t
Prevalite 28t
Prevnar 59t
PrevPac 53b
Priftin 18t
prilocaine 40b
Prilosec 55t
Primacor 34m
primaquine p 17m
Primaxin 20m
Primestrin 64b
primidone 61m
Primsol 25m
Principen 23m
Prinivil 25b
Prinzide 29b
Priscoline D
ProAmatine 34m
Pro-Banthine 55t
probenecid 44m
procainamide 27b
procaine peni 22b
Procanbid 27b
procarbazine 69t
Procardi 31b,67m
prochlorperaz 52b
crit 58m
dium 80b
Fast 76b
progester gel 68m
progesterone 67t
Progestins 66b
Proglycem 43m
Prograf 60m
proguanil 17m
ProHIBit 58b
Proleukin 69m
Prolixin 74m
Proloprim 25m
Promega 29t,45m
Pro-Meta 77m
promethazine 48m,49t,52b
Prometrium 67t
Pronestyl 27b
propafenone D
Propagest 49b
propantheline 55t
proparacaine 72t
Propecia 40b
Propine 71t
propofol 15m
propoxyphene 13b,13m,14b
propranolol 29m,31m
Propulsid 56m
propylene gly 50m
propylthioura 45b
Proscar 80m
Prosed/DS 81t
Prosobee 45m
ProSom 75t
prostaglandin D
Prostate canc 81b
Prostigmin 64t
Prostin VR Ped D
protamine 58m
Protease Inhi 19b
Protenate 35t
Proton pump i 55t
Protonix 55m
Protopam 80t
protriptyline D
Protropin 47t
Proventil 77m
Provera 66b
Provigil 76b
Provocholine D
Prozac 72m
pseudoephedrine 48b,48m,48t,49b
Psorcon 60,69
Psychiatry 70
psyllium 56t
PTU 45b
Pulmicort Tu 78m
Pulmonary 77
Pulmozyme 79t
Purge 55m
Purinethol 69m
Purinol 44t,81m
pyrantel 18m
pyrazina 17b,18t
pyrethrin 37b,37m
Pyridiate 80b
Pyridium 80b
pyridostigmin 64t
pyridoxine 46m
pyrilamine D
pyrimethami 18m
Pyronium 80b

Q

Quadramet 69b
Quelicin 16t
Questran 28t
quetiapine 74t
Quick-Pep 76m
Quinaglute 27b
Quinalan 27b
quinapril 25b,29m
Quinate 27b
Quinidex 27b
quinidine 27b
quinine sulfate 10t
Quinolones 23,24
Quinora 27b
quinupristin 25m

R

R&C Shamp 37m
RabAvert 58m
rabeprazole 55m
rabies im glob 60t
rabies vaccin 58m
rally pack 45m
raloxifene 67t
raloxifene 47t
ramipril 26t
ranitidine 53b
rapacuronium 15b
Rapamune 60m
Raplon 15b
rauwolfia D
Rauzide D
Reactine 47b
Rebetron D
Rebif 63b
Recombivax 58b
Refludan 58t
Regitine 30t
Reglan 52b
Regonal 64t
Regranex 40m
Relafen 11m
Relenza 20m
Relief 71b
Remeron 73m
Remicade 56m
remifentanil D
Remular-S 9b
Renagel 47t
Renedil 31b
Renese D
Renografin 35m
Renova 36t
ReoPro 30t
repaglinide 44t
Repronex 69t
Requip 63t
Rescriptor 19t
Resectisol 63b
reserpine 26b
RespiGam 60t
Restoril 75t
Retavase 34b
reteplase 34b
Retin-A 36t
Retisol-A 36t
Retrovir 19b
Reverse Trans 19
Reversol 63b
Revex 14b
ReVia 76t
Rheomacrode 35t
Rheumatrex 9m
Rhinalar 51m
Rhinocort Aqu 51t
Rhinocort 51t
RHO imm 60t,69t
RhoGAM 60t,69t
Rhotrimine D
ribavirin D
riboflavin 46m
RID 37b
Ridaura 9t
rifabutin 17b
Rifadin 17b,25t
Rifamate 17b
rifampin 17b,18t,25t
rifapentine 18t
Rifater 18t
Rilutek 64t
riluzole 64t
Rimactan 17b,25t
rimantadine 20m
rimexolone 70b
Riopan 53m
Riphenidate 76b
risedronate 41b
Risperdal 74t
risperidone 74t
Ritalin 76b
ritodrine 67m
ritonavir 20t
Rituxan 69m
rituximab 69m
rivastigmine 60b
Rivotril 60b,75t
rizatriptan 62t
Robaxin 9b
Robaxin-750 9b
Robaxisal 10m
Robitussin 48,49
Rocaltrol 46t
Rocephin 21m
rocuronium 16t
Rofact 17b,25t
rofecoxib 11b
Roferon-A 69m
Rogaine Forte 41t
Rogaine 41t
Rogitine 30t
Rolaids Calci 53t
Romazicon 79b
Rondec DM 48b
Rondec syrup 48b
ropinirole 63t
rosiglitazone 44t
Rowasa 56b
Roxanol 12b
Roxicet 14m
Roxicodone 13t
RSV imm glob 60t
Rubex 69m
Rufen 11t
Rylosol 28t
Rynatan P/S D
Rynatan 48b
Rynatan-12 S D
Rythmodan-LA D
Rythmol D

S

S.A.S. 9m
S-2 79m
IPOL 59t
Saizen 47t
Salazopyri 9m,57t
Salflex 11b
saline nasal s 51b
salmeterol 77b
salsalate 11b
Salutensin D
samarium 69b
Sandimmune 60t
Sandoglobuli 58b
Sandostatin 56b
SangCYA 60t
Sansert D
saquinavir 20t
Sarafem 77t
sargramosti 58m
scopolami 53t,54b
SeaMist 51b
Sea-Omega 29t
secobarbital D
Seconal D
Sectral 30b
Selective estr 67t
selegiline 63m

t = top of page
m = middle of page
b= bottom of page
D= for brevity in deluxe edition only

selenium sulfi 41t
Selpak 63m
Selsun 41t
Semprex-D D
senna 56t
Senokot 56t
Sensorcaine 15b
Septra 24t
Ser-A-Gen D
Ser-Ap-Es D
Serax 75t
Serentil D
Serevent 77b
Serophene 68b
Seroquel 74t
Serostim 47t
Serpasil 26b
Sertan 61m
sertraline 72b
Serzone 73m
sevelamer 47t
sexually trans21b
sibutramin57t,77t
sildenafil 81t
Silvadene 36m
silver sulfadi 36m
simethicone 53m,55t
Similac 45m
Simulect 60t
simvastatin 28b
Sinemet 63m
Sinequan 73t
Sinex 51m
Singulair 78b
sirolimus 60m
Skelaxin 9b
Skelid 41b
Slo-bid 78b
Slo-Phyllin 78b
SNRIs 72b
sodium ferric45m
sodium phos56m
sodium polyst47t
sodium sulfac35b
Solag 41t
Solaquin 40b
Solganal 9t
Solu-Cortef 42t
Solu-Medrol 42m,63b
Som Pam 74b
Soma wCod 14m
Soma Comp 10m
Soma 9b
Sominex 75m,77t
Somnol 74b
Somnote 75m
Sonata 75b
sorbitol 56m,80t
Sorbitrate 33m
Soriatane 37b
Sotacor 28t
sotalol 28t
Soyalac 45m
Spacol 80m
sparfloxacin 24t
Spasdel 80m
Spectazole 36b
spectinomycin D
spironolactone 29m,33t,47m
Sporanox 16b
SSRIs 72m
Stadol NS 12t
Stadol 12t
Starch 40t
Statex 12b
Statins 28m
stavudine 19b
Stay Awake 76m
Stelazine D
Stemetil 52b
Sterapred 42m
Stievaa 36t
Stimate 47t,58m
Stimulants 75m
Streptase 34b
streptokinase 34b
streptomycin D
streptozocin 69t
Stromectol 18t
strontium-89 69b
Sublimaze 15m
succimer 80t
succinylcholin 16t
sucralfate 55t
Sudafed 49b
Sufenta D
sufentanil D
Sulamyd 70t
Sular 32t
Sulf-10 70t
sulfacetamide 70t
Sulfacet-R 35b
sulfadiazine 24m
sulfamethoxazol 24m,24t
Sulfamylon 36t
sulfasalazi9m,57t
Sulfatrim 24t
sulfisoxazole 22m,24m
Sulfizole 24m
Sulfonamides 24t
Sulfonylureas42b
sulindac 11b
sumatriptan 62t
Sumycin 24b
SuperEPA 29t
Supeudol 13t
Suprax 21t
Surfak 55m
Surmontil D
Survanta D
Sustiva 19t
Sweet'n fresh 68t
Swim-Ear 50m
Symax 80m
Symmetrel20t,63t
Sympathomi 75m
Synacort 38,39
Synacthen 47t
Synagis D
Synalar 38,39
Synarel 65m
Synercid 25m
Synflex 11m
Synthroid 45b

T

T3, T4 45b
tacrine 60b
tacrolimus 60m
Tagamet 53m
Talacen 14m
Talwin 12t
Tambocor D
Tamiflu 20t
Tamofen 47m
Tamone 47m, 67t,69m
tamoxifen 47m, 67t,69m
tamsulosin 80m
Tapazole 45b
Tarka 29b
Tasmar 62b
Tavist 47b
Taxol 69m
Taxotere 69m
tazarotene36t,38t
Tazicef 21m
Tazidime 21m
Tazocin 23m
Tazorac 36t,38t
Td,DT 58b
TearsNaturale72t
Tebrazid 17b
Tegretol 60b,73b
Tegrin 40m
Tegrin-HC 38,39
telmisartan 26m
temazepam 75t
Temodar 69t
Temovate 38,39
temozolomide 69t
Tempra 15t
tenecteplase 34b
Tenex 77t
teniposide 69m
Tenoretic 29b
Tenormin 30b
Tensilon 63b
Tequin 24t
Teramine 76b
Terazol 68m
terazosi 26b,80m
terbinafine 17t,37m
terbutaline 67m,77b
terconazole 68m
Terfluzine D
Tessalon Per49m
Tes-Tape 43m
Testoderm 41m
testosterone 41m
Testred 41m
Testro AQ 41m
Testro-L.A. 41m
tetanus & per 58b
tetanus imm g60t
tetanus toxoi 58m
tetracaine 72t
tetracycline 24b,53b
Tetracyn 24b
Teveten 26t
Thalitone 33t
Theo-24 78b
Theo-Dur 78b
theophylline 78b
TheraCys 69m
thiabendazole D
thiamine 46m
thiethylperazineD
thioguanine 69m
thiopental 15m
Thioplex 69t
thioridazine 74b
thiotepa 69t
thiothixene D
thonzium 50t
Thorazine 74m
Thrombolytics34b
Thyro-Block D
thyroid - dessic D
Thyroid Agents45b
Thyroid USP D
Thyrolar 45b
tiagabine 61b
Tiamate 32t
Tiazac 32t
Ticar 23m
ticarcillin clav23m
ticarcillin 23m
Tice BCG Va69m
Tice BCG 58b
Ticlid 30b
ticlopidine 30b
Tigan 53t
Tikosyn 27m
Tilade 79m
tiludronate 41b
Timentin 23m
Timolide 29b
timolol 29b, 31m,70b,71t
Timoptic XE 70b
Timoptic 70b
Tinactin 37m
tinzaparin 57b
tioconazole 68b
tirofiban 30b
Titralac 53t
tizanidine 10t
TNKase 34b
TOBI 16t
TobraDex 70b
tobramycin 16t, 70b,70t
Tobrex 70t
tocainide D
Tocolytics 67m
tocopherol 46b
Tofranil 73t,80b
Tofranil-PM 80b
tolazamide D
tolazoline D
tolbutamide D
tolcapone 62b
Tolectin 12t
Tolinase D
tolmetin 12t
tolnaftate 37m
Tol-Tab D
tolterodine 81t
Tonocard D
Topactin 38,39
Topamax 61b
topical 38b
Topicort LP38,39
Topicort 38,39
topiramate 61b
Topisone 38,39
Toposar 69m
topotecan 69m
Toprol XL 31m
Toradol 11m
Torecan D
toremifene 69m
Tornalate 77m
torsemide 32b
Toxicology 79
t-PA 34b,63m
tramadol 15t
Trandate 31t

t = top of page
m = middle of page
b= bottom of page
D= for brevity in deluxe edition only

trandolapr26t,29b
TransdermSc 53t
*TransdermNitr*34t
Transderm-V 53t
Tranxene D
tranylcypromineD
trastuzumab 69m
Travel Tabs 49t
trazodone 73m
Trazorel 73m
Trecator-SC 17b
Tremytoine 61m
Trental 58m
tretinoin 36t,41t,69b
Triacin-C 48b
Triadapin 73t
triamcinolone 38,39,42m, 50b,51b,78b
Triaminic 48b
*Triaminic Infa*49b
triamtere29b,29m
Triavil D
triazolam 75m
trichlormethiazi D
Tricor 28b
Tridesilon 38,39
Tridil 33b
triethanolami50m
trifluoperazine D
trifluridine 70m
trihexyphenid62b
TriHibit 58m
*Trikacide*18m,25t
Trilafon D
Trileptal 61m
Tri-Levlen 65
Trilisate 12t
trimacinolone38m
trimethaphan D
trimethobenza53t
trimethoprim 24t,25m,70t
trimipramine D
Trimox 23t
Tri Nasal 61b
Trinipatch 34t
Tri-Norinyl 65
Tripedia 58b
Triphasil 65
olidine48b,48t
til D
c 53b
Trivora-28 65
Trobicin D
tropicamide 71b
trovafloxacin 24t
Trovan 24t
Trusopt 71t
*Truxadryl*75m,77t
tuberculin 60m
Tubersol 60m
Tucks 40t
Tuinal D
Tums 53t
Tuss-HC 48b
Tusstat 75m,77t
Tylenol Cod 14m
Tylenol 15t
Tylox 14m
Typhim Vi 58m
typhoid vacci58m

U

Ultiva D
Ultradol 10b
Ultram 15t
Ultravate 38,39
Unasyn 23m
Uni-Decon 48b
Uni-Dur 78b
Uniphyl 78b
Uniretic 29b
*Unisom Nigh*52m
Univasc 25b
Urecholine 81m
Urex D
Urised 81t
Urispas 80m
Urocit-K 81m
Urodol 80b
Urogesic 80b
urokinase D
*Urolene b*80t,81m
Urology 80
Urso 57m
ursodiol 57m
Ursofalk 57m
Uterotonics 67b
UTI Relief 80b

V

Vagifem 68t
Vaginal Preps67b
vaginitis 21b
Vagistat-1 68b
valacyclovir 19t
Valergen 20 64m
Valergen 40 64m
*Valium*9b,60b,75t
valproic acid 61b,62m,73b
valrubicin 69m
valsartan 26m,29m
Valstar 69m
Valtrex 19t
Vanatrip 72b
Vancenase 51t
Vanceril 78m
Vancocin 25m
vancomycin 25m
Vantin 21t
Vaqta 58b
varicella vacc58m
varicella im gl 60t
Varivax 58m
Vascor D
Vaseretic 29b
Vasocon 72t
Vasodilan D
vasopressin 47m,57m
Vasotec 25b
Vasoxyl D
Vaxigrip 59t
VCR 69b
vecuronium 16t
Veetids 22b
Velban 69m
venlafaxine 73t
Venoglobulin 58b
Ventodisk 77m
Ventolin 77m
VePesid 69m
verapam29b,32m
Verelan PM 32m
Vermox 18m
Versed 15m,75t
Versel 41t
verteporfin D
Vesanoid 69b
Vexol 70b
Viactiv 53t
Viagra 81t
Vibramycin 17m,24m,35b
Vibra-Tabs 17m
Vick's 49m
Vicodin 14m
Vicoprofen 14b
vidarabine 70m
Videx 19m
vinblastine 69m
Vincasar 69b
vincristine 69b
vinorelbine 69b
Viokase 57t
Vioxx 11b
Vira-A 70m
Viracept 20t
Viramune 19m
Virazole D
Virilon IM 41m
Virilon 41m
Viroptic 70m
Visken 31m
Vistaril 49t
Vistide 18b
Visudyne D
vitamin B1 46m
vitamin B12 46t
vitamin B2 46m
*vitami B3*29t,46m
vitamin B6 46m
vitamin C 46t
vitamin D 46t
vitamin E 46b
vitamin K 46m
Vitamins 46t
Vitravene D
Vivactil D
Vivarin 76m
Vivelle Dot 64m
Vivelle 64m
Vivol 60b,75t
Vivotif Berna 58m
VLB 69m
Vofenal 71b
Volmax 77m
Voltaren XR 10b
Voltaren 10b,71b
VoSol otic 50m
VP-16 69m
Vumon 69m
VZIG 60t

W

warfarin 58t
Warfilone 58t
Welchol 28t
Wellbutrin 73m
Westcort 38,39
Wigraine 62m
Winpred 42m
WinRho SDF 60t
witch hazel 40t
Wyamine D
Wycillin 22b
Wygesic 14b
Wytensin D

X

Xalatan 71m
Xanax 74b
Xeloda 69m
Xenical 57t
Xopenex 77m
Xylocaine 15b, 27m,40b,50b
Xylocard 27m

Y

yellow fever 58m
YF-Vax 58m
Yodoxin D
Yutopar 67m

Z

Zaditor 71b
zafirlukast 78b
Zagam 24t
zalcitabine 19b
zaleplon 75b
Zanaflex 10t
zanamivir 20m
Zanosar 69t
Zantac 75 53b
Zantac 53b
Zapex 75t
Zarontin 61t
Zaroxolyn 33m
ZDV 19b
Zebeta 31t
Zemplar 46m
Zemuron 16t
Zenapax 60t
Zephrex-LA 48b
Zerit 19b
Zestoretic 29b
Zestril 25b
Ziac 29b
Ziagen 19m
zidovudine 19bm
zileuton 78b
Zinacef 20b
zinc oxide 40t
Zithromax 22t
Zocor 28b
Zofran 52m
Zoladex 64b, 69m,81b
zolmitriptan 62t
Zoloft 72b
zolpidem 75b
Zomig 62t
Zonalon 40m,73t
Zonegran 61b
zonisamide 61b
Zostrix 40m
Zostrix-HP 40m
Zosyn 23m
Zovia 65
Zovirax 18b,38t
Zyban 75b
Zydone 14b
Zyflo 78b
Zyloprim 44t,81m
Zyprexa 74t
Zyrtec 47b
Zyvox 25t

Page left blank for notes

Page left blank for notes

ADULT EMERGENCY DRUGS (selected)

ALLERGY	cimetidine (*Tagamet*). 300 mg IV/IM. diphenhydramine (*Benadryl*): 50 mg IV/IM. epinephrine: 0.1-0.5 mg SC (1:1000 solution), may repeat after 20 minutes. methylprednisolone (*Solu-Medrol*): 125 mg IV/IM.
DYSRHYTHMIAS / CARDIAC ARREST	adenosine (*Adenocard*): SVT (not A-fib/flutter): 6 mg rapid IV & flush, preferably through a central line. If no response after 1-2 minutes then 12 mg. A third dose of 12-18 mg may be given prn. atropine: 0.5-1.0 mg IV/ET. bretylium (*Bretylol*): Initial 5 mg/kg IV, repeat 10 mg/kg if needed. Infusion 500 mg in 50ml D5W (10 mg/ml) at 1-3 mg/min (7-21 ml/h). diltiazem (*Cardizem*): Rapid atrial fibrillation: bolus 0.25 mg/kg or 20 mg IV over 2 min. Infusion 5-15 mg/h. epinephrine: 1 mg IV/ET for cardiac arrest. [1:10,000 solution] lidocaine (*Xylocaine*): Load 1 mg/kg IV, then 0.5 mg/kg q8-10min as needed to max 3 mg/kg. Maintenance 2g in 250ml D5W (8 mg/ml) at 1-4 mg/min drip (7-30 ml/h). procainamide (*Pronestyl*): 100 mg IV q10min or run infusion below at 20 mg/min (150 ml/h) until: 1) QRS or PR widens >50%, 2) Dysrhythmia suppressed, 3) Hypotension, or 4) Total of 17 mg/kg or 1000 mg. Infusion 2g in 250ml D5W (8 mg/ml) at 2-6 mg/min (15-45 ml/h).
PRESSORS	dobutamine (*Dobutrex*). 250 mg in 250ml D5W (1 mg/ml) at 2.5-15 mcg/kg/min. 70 kg: 21 ml/h = 5 mcg/kg/min. dopamine (*Intropin*). 400 mg in 250ml D5W (1600 mcg/ml) at 2-20 mcg/kg/min. 70 kg: 13 ml/h = 5 mcg/kg/min. Doses in mcg/kg/min: 2-5 = dopaminergic, 5-10 = beta, >10 = alpha. norepinephrine (*Levophed*): 4 mg in 500 ml D5W (8 mcg/ml) at 2-4 mcg/min. 20 ml/h = 3 mcg/min. phenylephrine (*Neo-Synephrine*): 50 mcg boluses IV. Infusion for hypotension: 20 mg in 250ml D5W (80 mcg/ml) at 40-180 mcg/min (35-160ml/h).
INTUBATION	etomidate (*Amidate*): 0.3 mg/kg IV. methohexital (*Brevital*): 1-1.5 mg/kg IV. rocuronium (*Zemuron*): 0.6-1.2 mg/kg IV. succinylcholine (*Anectine*): 1 mg/kg IV. Peds (<5 yo): 2 mg/kg IV preceded by atropine 0.02 mg/kg. thiopental (*Pentothal*): 3-5 mg/kg IV.
SEIZURES	diazepam (*Valium*): 5-10 mg IV, or 0.2-0.5 mg/kg rectal gel up to 20 mg PR. fosphenytoin (*Cerebyx*): Load 15-20 "phenytoin equivalents" per kg either IM, or IV no faster than 100-150 mg/min. lorazepam (*Ativan*): 0.05-0.15 mg/kg up to 3-4 mg IV/IM magnesium sulfate: Eclampsia: 1-4 g IV over 2-4 min. phenobarbital: 200- 600 mg IV at rate ≤60 mg/min up to 20 mg/kg. phenytoin (*Dilantin*): Load 15-20 mg/kg up to 1000 mg IV no faster than 50 mg/min.

CARDIAC DYSRHYTHMIA PROTOCOLS

Basic Life Support

All cases: Two initial breaths, then compressions 80-100 per minute
One rescuer: 15:2 ratio of compressions to ventilations
Two rescuer or Pediatric: 5:1 ratio of compressions to ventilations

V-Fib, Pulseless V-Tach

CPR until defibrillator ready
Defibrillate 200 J
Defibrillate 200-300 J
Defibrillate 360 J
Intubate, IV
Epinephrine 1 mg IV/ET q3-5 minutes
Defibrillate 360 J after each drug dose
Options:
Lidocaine 1.5 mg/kg IV q3-5 minutes to max 3 mg/kg
Bretylium 5 mg/kg IV
Magnesium 1-2 g IV
Procainamide 30 mg/min IV to max 17 mg/kg
Bicarbonate 1 meq/kg IV

Stable Ventricular Tachycardia

Airway, oxygen, IV
Lidocaine 1-1.5 mg/kg IV
Lidocaine 0.5-0.75 mg/kg IV q5-10 min to total 3 mg/kg
Procainamide 20-30 mg/min to max 17 mg/kg
Bretylium 5-10 mg/kg over 8-10 min
Consider cardioversion

Stable Wide-Complex Tachycardia

Airway, oxygen, IV
Lidocaine 1-1.5 mg/kg IV
Lidocaine 0.5-0.75 mg/kg IV q5-10 min to total 3 mg/kg
Adenosine 6 mg rapid IV, wait 1-2 min
Adenosine 12 mg rapid IV, wait 1-2 min
Adenosine 12 mg rapid IV, wait 1-2 min
Procainamide 20-30 mg/min IV to max 17 mg/kg
Bretylium 5-10 mg/kg IV over 8-10 min
Consider cardioversion

Pulseless Electrical Activity (EMD)

CPR, intubate, IV
Consider hypovolemia, hypoxia, cardiac tamponade, tension pneumothorax, hypothermia, massive PE, drug OD, hyperkalemia, acidosis, massive MI
Epinephrine 1 mg IV/ET q3-5 minutes
Atropine 1 mg IV if heart rate <60/min

Asystole

CPR, intubate, IV
Confirm asystole in >1 lead
Consider hypoxia, hyperkalemia, hypokalemia, preexisting acidosis, drug OD, hypothermia
Consider external pacing
Epinephrine 1 mg IV/ET q3-5 minutes
Atropine 1 mg IV/ET, repeat in 3-5 min

Bradycardia (<60), symptomatic

Airway, oxygen, IV
Atropine 0.5-1 mg IV q3-5 min up to 2 mg total
External pacemaker
Options: Dopamine 5-20 mcg/kg/min
Epinephrine 2-10 mcg/min
Consider Isoproterenol

Unstable Tachycardia (>150/min)

Airway, oxygen, IV
Consider brief trial of medications
Consider cardioversion sedation
Synchronized cardioversion 100 J
Synchronized cardioversion 200 J
Synchronized cardioversion 300 J
Synchronized cardioversion 360 J

Stable PSVT

Airway, oxygen, IV
Vagal maneuvers
Adenosine 6 mg rapid IV, wait 1-2 min
Adenosine 12 mg rapid IV, wait 1-2 min
Adenosine 18 mg rapid IV, wait 1-2 min
If narrow complex, consider verapamil, digoxin, β-blockers, or diltiazem,
If wide complex, consider lidocaine or procainamide
Consider cardioversion

Ordering Books From Tarascon Publishing

FAX	PHONE	INTERNET	MAIL
Fax orders with credit card info 24 hours/day to **877.929.9926**	For phone orders or customer service, call **800.929.9926**	Order through our OnLine store with your credit card at **www.tarascon.com**	Mail order & check to: **Tarascon Publishing PO Box 1159 Loma Linda, CA 92354**

Name

Address

City | State | Zip

Please send me:	*Quantity*	*Price (table)*
Tarascon Pocket Pharmacopoeia, 2001 Classic Edition		$
Tarascon Pocket Pharmacopoeia, 2001 Deluxe Edition		$
Tarascon Internal Med & Critical Care Pocketbk, 2nd ed		$
How to be a Truly Excellent Junior Medical Student, 6th ed		$
Tarascon Adult Emergency Pocketbook, 1st ed		$
Tarascon Pediatric Emergency Pocketbook, 3rd ed		$

Price per Copy by Number of Each Title Ordered

Total # each ordered	1–9	10–49	50-99	≥100
Pocket Pharm, Classic	$7.95	$6.95	$5.95	$5.55
Pocket Pharm, Deluxe	$17.95	$15.25	$13.45	$12.55
Internal Med Pocketbk	$11.95	$9.90	$8.95	$8.35
Excellent Junior Med	$9.95	$8.25	$7.45	$6.95
Adult Emerg Pocketbk	$9.95	$8.25	$7.45	$6.95
Peds Emerg Pocketbk	$9.95	$8.25	$7.45	$6.95

Subtotal	$
In CA only: add 7.75% Sales Tax	$
Shipping & handling (see table)	$
TOTAL	$

Shipping & Handling

If subtotal is →	<$10	$10-24	$25-109	$110-400
Standard shipping	$1.00	$2.50	$4.00	$8.00
UPS 2-day air*	$10.00	$10.00	$12.50	$15.00

**No post office boxes*

❒ **Charge credit card:** ❒ VISA ❒ Mastercard ❒ American Express

Card number | Exp Date

Signature | E-mail | Phone